Leadership with Compassion:

Applying Kindness, Dignity and Respect in Healthcare Management

Clive Lewis OBE DL

Copyright © 2013 by Clive Lewis

First published in Great Britain in 2013

By

Globis Ltd
Unit 1
Wheatstone Court
Waterwells Business Park
Quedgeley
Gloucester
GL2 2AQ

The right of Clive Lewis to be identified as the Author of the Work has been asserted by him in accordance with the Copyright, Designs and Patents Act 1988.

All rights reserved. No part of this publication may be reproduced, stored in a retrievable system, or transmitted, in any form or by any means without the prior written consent of the Author, nor be otherwise circulated in any form of binding or cover other than that in which it is published and without a similar condition being imposed on the subsequent purchaser.

ISBN 978-0-9575246-0-6

Cover design by Brendan Vaughan-Spruce

Printed and bound in the UK by:

**Berforts Information Press
23-35 Gunnels Wood Park
Stevenage
Hertfordshire
SG1 2BH**

Also by the author

The Definitive Guide to Workplace Mediation and Managing Conflict at Work

Win Win – Resolving Workplace Conflict

Workplace Mediation Skills – Training Handbook

Difficult Conversations – 10 Steps to Becoming a Tackler not a Dodger

Difficult Conversations in Dementia – A Ten Step Toolkit for Clinicians Involved in End of Life Discussions

Bouncing Back from Redundancy – 12 Steps to Get Your Career and Life Back on Track

Work-Life Balance – How to Put Work in its Place and Reclaim Your Life

Performance Management – Ten Steps to Getting the Most from Your Workforce

Contents

Introduction	1
Chapter One: Acknowledge and address	7
Chapter Two: Professional is personal	14
Chapter Three: Make it a habit	23
Chapter Four: Be inspired	33
Chapter Five: Take time out	42
Chapter Six: Get a fresh perspective	51
Chapter Seven: Keeping it real	60
Chapter Eight: Respect begins at home	67

Chapter Nine: Actions speak loudest	75
Chapter Ten: Patients as customers	82
Chapter Eleven: Culture shift	92
Chapter Twelve: A note on saying sorry	100
Chapter Thirteen: Keep at it!	106
Conclusion	113
About the author	114
Order form	115
References	116

Introduction

The UK healthcare system is under the microscope. It is experiencing what could be described as a 'care crisis'. Several high profile inquiries have revealed shockingly poor quality of care in hospitals, residential homes and other healthcare settings. But what has really happened? Have nurses, midwives and doctors suddenly stopped caring? Are we recruiting care assistants who are missing a compassion gene? Probably not. The majority of people working within the healthcare sector start their careers intending to look after their patients to the best of their ability. We should be asking what it is that is preventing some people from demonstrating this care in their daily work.

The Department of Health has set out a series of recommendations and initiatives that it believes will restore public confidence in the caring professions. It has coined the term 'The Six Cs' to describe the personal qualities all healthcare professionals should have. These are:

Care   Compassion

Competence   Communication

Courage   Commitment

The UK healthcare system is in the midst of what could be called a 'care crisis'.

This is probably not due to a deficiency in compassion by healthcare staff, but we should be asking why some people are being prevented from demonstrating care in their work.

The Department of Health has set out 'The Six Cs' to describe the personal qualities all healthcare professionals should have:

*Care
Compassion
Competence
Communication
Courage
Commitment*

Readers who engage with the contents of this book and the exercises in each chapter should discover that they have improved their skills in each 'C' by the end.

Readers should find that their skills in each 'C' have improved by the end of this book.

Who is this handbook for?

If you manage a team or department within the NHS or private healthcare sector then this book is for you. We will address issues that will improve your ability to manage your team, enhance their performance and enable them to treat their patients with the dignity and respect they deserve. The exercises at the end of each chapter will help you to improve your relationships with your board and senior management team as well as those you line manage. They will even have a positive impact on your personal life if you choose to adopt the techniques at home as well as at work.

This handbook is for those who manage a team or department within both the private and public healthcare sectors.

Engaging with this book and the exercises at the end of each chapter will improve not only your professional life but your personal life as well.

Why I wrote Leadership with Compassion

There are a number of reasons why I have written this handbook, four of which I will briefly outline here.

A few years ago my father died of renal failure, a loss that devastated our family. We were able to share our grief with Dr. Williams, the consultant who had treated him over the previous five years. Not only was Dr. Williams highly experienced and knowledgeable, he also understood the importance of communication with the

This book takes its inspiration from a number of sources, one of which was the death of my father.

patient *and* their family. He made sure my mother was kept up to date with the latest news about my father's condition and made time for them both at appointments. He made the effort when my father was admitted to hospital to go up to his ward and check on his progress, even though he wasn't involved in his care at that late stage. He considered the patient as a whole person rather than simply seeing their condition, and was skilled at delivering bad news. I can vividly recall one occasion when he called the family together. He wanted to tell us that my father's blood circulation was poor and as a result it was only a matter of time before he would lose his left foot. A similar gathering took place at a later stage in my father's illness when Dr. Williams broke the news to the family that my father's condition was worsening and that we should begin to prepare for life without him. He eventually passed away a few days after my son's christening service which was held in the hospital chapel so that my father could attend. The humane way Dr. Williams treated me and my family is something for which I will be eternally grateful – he made a very difficult and painful situation easier to live with.

Secondly, I am frequently called upon to mediate disputes or negotiate situations within the healthcare

The doctor looking after my father was excellent.

He kept my mother informed every step of the way, made time for them both at appointments and even visited my father in hospital when he was no longer involved in his care. He was also skilled in delivering bad news.

He treated not just the condition or the patient, rather the whole person and all that came with that commitment.

The humane way in which he treated not only my father but also our family made a very difficult and painful time easier to live with.

sector. I remember one dispute between two doctors which thankfully ended with a satisfactory conclusion for both involved, but an unfortunate part to their story has stayed with me. The fall out related to some treatment administered to a patient by one of the doctors; the patient's notes indicated that he was allergic to morphine, but somehow the doctor responsible for his care on a particular day gave the patient morphine. The effect was devastating – on a short tip to the lavatory, shortly after receiving the treatment, the patient lost his balance and fell. The impact knocked his teeth through his lip and blackened his eyes. This is the lasting memory his wife and children have of their loved one who died a few days afterwards. The doctor who didn't administer the lethal dosage was angry with her colleague for what happened.

Whilst this part of the story is disturbing, there was a further part which also struck me. The doctor responsible desperately wanted to meet with the family and offer her apology and support, but the internal grievance procedure prevented the doctor from having any contact with the family, thus preventing such a conversation from taking place. This was very unfortunate and didn't make much sense to me.

I also frequently mediate on disputes or negotiations in the healthcare sector.

One case involved a doctor who had accidentally given a patient morphine who was allergic to it. The patient collapsed shortly afterwards and died several days later.

The doctor responsible desperately wanted to apologise to the family face to face, but the formal grievance procedure didn't allow for that.

This situation didn't make sense to me and prevented a level of emotional healing for both parties.

Eighteen months of anguish through a grievance process could have been prevented. Perhaps a seventh C should be 'Common sense'.

Third, as a non-executive director in the NHS, I am made aware of a number of incidents ranging from serious untoward incidents (SUIs) to surgery appointments that are cancelled on the day of delivery. It strikes me that the role of the apology could play a far more important role in the life of the healthcare organisation. Research has been conducted on this theme, more of which I will touch on in Chapter Eleven, but I am keen to hear from readers to whom this suggestion appeals. It only takes a few people with an idea and passion to create change.

Fourth and finally, I would like to talk about Maggie, a nursing director on the board of an NHS Foundation Trust I work with. She began her healthcare career on the wards and although she has worked her way up the management ladder she has not lost any of her passion for providing excellent care. She talks with great enthusiasm about infection control and is open and honest about learning from mistakes. She has supported the process of inviting patients/their families to board meetings in order to provide feedback about the care they received. Maggie is completely patient-

Perhaps a seventh 'C' should be 'Common sense'.

As a non-executive director in the NHS I am made aware of a number of incidents ranging from serious incidents to last minute surgery cancellations.

I am convinced that the apology could play a major role in situations such as this, and would like to hear from others who feel the same way.

I occasionally work with a nursing director, Maggie, who worked her way up from the hospital ward to the boardroom without losing her passion for providing excellent care.

She has supported strategies promoting communication and openness between patients/their families and board members, in order that they receive direct feedback.

centred and still manages to be highly effective in the management of her teams. I am inspired by what I see both with her and in her.

My experiences of being with Dr. Williams and Maggie (in completely different capacities) have shown me how important it is for senior healthcare staff to lead with compassion. They understand that good care is not optional or 'nice to have' and that making respect for the patient central to their decisions has made them more effective managers and clinicians.

These various experiences have illustrated to me the importance of senior staff leading with compassion.

Good care should not be optional but a foundation on which to build.

I don't believe you can 'make' people care or be more compassionate. But, you can enhance your own ability to be the most caring person you can be, removing obstacles (be they emotional or practical) along the way. It doesn't matter if you don't complete all of the exercises (although the more you do the more effective this programme will be for you). We're all different, and you will be more drawn to some subject areas than others. But I do ask that you begin this journey with an open heart and mind. It is my intention that at the end of this book you will have a renewed enthusiasm for working in healthcare and feel confident that you have the tools to be the a highly compassionate *and* effective manager.

I don't believe you can make people care, but you can teach yourself how to be the most caring person you can be, which, in turn, may inspire others in the way I have been inspired.

Clive Lewis

Chapter One: Acknowledge and address

"We have a problem". How do you react when you hear that statement? It depends on the context, of course. If it's your manager speaking, you may immediately think of something that didn't go to plan or that you hoped they wouldn't notice. If it's your employee, you may be imagining possible scenarios involving resignation, misconduct, or personal difficulties. If it's your spouse, you could be anticipating an announcement of illness, infidelity or the DIY shop running out of Superglue (depending on the state of your relationship and whether or not your partner has a flair for the dramatic).

The words "We have a problem" can stir different emotions within us, depending on the context and the person informing us.

In all of these scenarios however, the most common feeling you're likely to experience is fear – fear of blame, of repercussions or of loss (be it loss of status, approval, or of a person). It may even be fear of change itself. Fear can keep us stuck in undesirable situations because we don't know how to act.

The most common emotion however is fear – fear of blame, of repercussions or of loss. It may even be fear of change itself. Fear often prevents action.

All too often we do nothing. We minimise or deny that there is a problem at all ("she's just having an off day", "it's not such a big deal, everyone else does it", or "it's just the way the world works"). All of these statements may be true, but they should only be concluded after

We often minimise the problem or deny that there is a problem at all.

we have looked the problem square in the face. We live in such a solution-focused culture that we can often spend far too little time thinking about the issue in hand and fast forward straight to the various options. Only by properly naming and identifying the problem can we begin the journey towards change.

We regularly afford too much time to the solution of a problem at the expense of identifying the root cause.

In Alcoholics Anonymous and other 12-step programmes, the first step is to admit the problem and the fact that life has become 'unmanageable' as a result. Only then can the person following the programme take the other steps towards recovery. This makes sense in the world of work as well – you can't change a situation or a person until you really understand what you're trying to change. Why, then, are so many organisations (and individuals) so loath to own up to problems?

Admission of a problem is commonly held as the first step to resolving it, particularly so with associations involved in eradicating addictions.

This is also true in the world of work, but many organisations (and individuals) are loath to own up to problems.

For companies, upsetting investors may affect their share price and tarnish their reputation. In the public sector, senior managers can be afraid to admit to problems for fear of discrediting politicians and facing accusations of wasting taxpayers' money.

Companies risk negatively affecting share prices or tarnishing reputations if they admit failure, and senior managers of public bodies can be accused of wasting taxpayers' money if they do the same.

Too often, bad practice is hidden through fear of exposure and blame and yet, in the end, it nearly always comes to light. This may take the form of whistleblowing or exposure by an investigation (by the

Bad practice often remains hidden, often only revealed through investigation (by external or internal agencies), which makes things worse.

authorities or the media). Often it is only at this point that change occurs, but at that stage you are on the back foot. By 'feeling the fear' and taking ownership of a problem as soon as it arises, you have in your possession something very valuable: control.

Taking ownership of a problem as soon as it arises ensures that you retain control of it.

We currently have a problem with compassion within our healthcare system, an area in which the NHS is investing millions of pounds. Tens of thousands of people leading teams are set to undergo training in compassion in an attempt to reverse the current situation, where overstretched and target-driven managers put such 'soft' qualities as respect a long way down on their list of priorities, often despite the best of intentions.

The NHS is investing millions of pounds in improving compassion among its staff.

Recent changes have seen targets put above compassion.

It is not within the remit of this book however to point fingers at the system and draw up suggestions for institutional change. My objective is to identify what we, as leaders in the healthcare sector, can do to effect positive change within our own environment. And I believe that starts with changing ourselves.

My objective however is to identify what we as healthcare leaders can do to effect positive change within our own environment. I believe such change starts with ourselves.

If you are committed to improving care within your team (and wider organisation) you need to have the courage to acknowledge the current state of play. Honesty is essential. To this end, you need to choose a dedicated space for dealing with the situation, not a

To work through the exercises in this book you need a dedicated, personal space, such as a computer or tablet, but ensure that they are not shared or work devices. I prefer a pen and notepad.

shared computer or company laptop. You can use a personal tablet, computer or phone, but I actually prefer to use a pen and paper. This way you can jot things down as you go along – plus it's also harder to self-censor without a delete button. We will be doing exercises throughout the book that require some powerful self-reflection, so make sure you have plenty of space (both physical and mental) to approach the task.

Ensure that you have enough space, both physical and mental, to approach the task.

How 'official' you make it is up to you. Initially, you may choose to focus on your own interactions with your team and observe their behaviour with their own patients. Depending on the level of support you have from senior management, you might wish to undertake an official 'care audit' involving anonymous staff surveys and questions in appraisals. However, I would suggest keeping your efforts informal and personal at first, because a) in some organisations you might be warned against engaging in such activities before you even start and b) if you are successful with your own 'compassion plan', it can be easier to convince senior managers when you have some evidence of success. A lot of companies can be risk-averse (fearing internal and external criticism), so carrying out your own care audit initially is a good place to start.

How 'official' you make it is up to you. Depending on your relationship with senior management you may wish to undertake an official 'care audit', or you might prefer to keep it personal.

I would advise keeping it personal at first and then approaching others if you meet with success.

Give yourself an hour and write down everything that comes to mind when you think about compassion and care. At this stage it doesn't matter whether you're thinking large or small, but try and get it all down. You may like to organise your thoughts under the headings of 'where it works' and 'where it doesn't'. It can be easy to focus simply on what's wrong, but it's also important to acknowledge good examples of care because there may be useful lessons to learn or skills to transfer from existing practices.

Once you have everything written down, you can organise your headings into themes or subject areas such as 'team relationships', 'personal development', 'reporting structure', 'workload', etc.

With a broad overview of how things are, you can begin to tackle areas for change. It can be a relief not to hide or justify poor practice any longer. Now you have shone a light on the good, the bad and the ugly, you can create a plan for change. How you go about this is up to you. You can start small and identify quick wins (such as extending your face to face meetings with staff by ten minutes to allow time for non-work related discussion), or you can choose one big area and focus all your energies on it. But choose something where you can take a practical step towards positive change and do

Give yourself an hour and write down everything that comes to mind when you think about compassion and care.

You may like to organise your thoughts under the headings of 'where it works' and 'where it doesn't'.

Ensure you don't simply focus on what's wrong but acknowledge good examples of care.

Organise your headings into themes or subject areas such as 'team relationships', 'personal development', 'reporting structure', 'workload', etc.

You can begin to tackle areas for change in whichever manner you choose, either identifying several quick wins or one large area of change.

Ensure you choose areas where practical positive steps are possible and do something about it every day.

something about it every day. The cumulative impact of your actions and decisions can have significant and far-reaching positive effects.

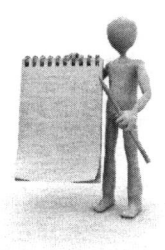

Exercises

Buy a notebook for your 'care project', or use a piece of technology that you know will not be seen by anyone else.

Write down a summary of your current situation. This can include any concerns you have, incidents that have occurred, and what led you to seek out this book.

Draw up some goals for your project. Try and make them as specific as possible, e.g. "I would like to receive some positive feedback from patients about my team's care and compassion" rather than just "I want to make my organisation a more caring and respectful place". There's nothing wrong with the latter, but it can be hard to know where to start when faced with such a general objective.

"The first step towards change is awareness. The second step is acceptance."

Nathaniel Branden

"Great leadership does not mean running away from reality."

John Kotter

"A problem is a chance for you to do your best."

Duke Ellington

Chapter Two: Professional is personal

As babies and young children, we are unafraid of expressing our wants and needs. If we want food, a cuddle or a change, we cry. We are the centre of our worlds, and this is just as it should be.

As we grow older, our parents and other authority figures begin to shape our behaviour. They ask us to share, to not hit other children, and to ask nicely for the things we want. This is the beginning of empathy and of learning to acknowledge other people's feelings. Nice behaviour is rewarded, aggressive or disobedient behaviour gets you sent straight to the naughty step.

As we grow older, our wants are diluted as we are taught to think of others.

But somewhere along the line, the message is subverted. 'Nice' may be all well and good, 'gentle' may get you friends, but it will not help you reach targets, discipline underperforming staff or to broker a deal. The aphorism that "nice guys finish last" might have been coined by a baseball team manager in the 1930s, but it came to prominence in the 1980s when the onus was on making as much money as possible, regardless of the consequences for others. Conspicuous capitalism was rife, and the UK was governed by its first female prime minister whose nickname 'the Iron Lady'

This message gets confused somewhere along the line however – we are told that "nice" doesn't meet targets or help discipline staff.

This message was reinforced more than ever in the capitalism boom of the 1980s, where ruthlessness was richly rewarded.

epitomised the harsh and self-serving ethos of the decade.

Fast forward to the late 1990s and a new system of values was welcomed into the workplace. With it came an influx of consultants who were paid extortionate sums to engage in lengthy team building exercises. When applying for jobs you needed to show exactly why your 'interpersonal strengths' (a term that only became popular relatively recently) matched your experience and qualifications. 'Soft' skills were all the rage.

So, however, were targets. Performance-related pay entered the business lexicon and managers and their employees approached appraisal time with trepidation. Were they good enough? What would happen if they didn't reach their targets? SMART goals were all very well, but they were (and remain) a blunt instrument for assessing performance in the round.

As the world economy has shrunk, people are being asked to do more with less. The targets remain the same, but there are fewer resources allocated to meeting them. This means that managers are under increasing pressure to deliver results, and they need their teams to be working at full steam. Soft skills? No

In the late 1990s a new system of values was welcomed into the workplace, where 'soft' skills and interpersonal strengths were lauded and sought after.

Targets and performance related pay became more prevalent too, with employees quickly beginning to fear appraisal time.

The worldwide financial crisis has left companies needing to achieve more with fewer resources.

Once more, soft skills are out – jobs need doing and they need doing now.

time for that, the job needs doing and it needs to be done NOW!

Sound familiar? You may view personal attributes such as being caring or generous as ideal rather than essential, but the evidence overwhelmingly shows that being kind and caring towards your staff and customers is good for morale *and* productivity. You don't have to take your team on paintballing weekends to show your human side. Reaching out where you can, appreciating the strengths of others and treating them as individuals with feelings can improve performance drastically.

Just look at some of the organisations at the top of the Sunday Times 100 Best Companies to Work For[1]. Yes, they are private companies who can take some liberties with what they offer their staff (e.g. the number one company offers very flexible working and benefits, finding out what each employee would do if they were managing director, offering a personal development fund and a month long sabbatical after five years of service). But their ultimate concern will still be the bottom line – they have a major financial interest in keeping people happy.

Whether we operate in the public or private sector, we all have to deliver value for money. But when people work for a boss who is genuinely interested in their

If this scenario feels familiar, consider the notion that being kind and caring towards your staff increases morale and productivity, backed up by a growing body of evidence.

A large number of the Sunday Times 100 Best Companies to Work For place great emphasis on staff morale whilst also managing to keep the books healthy.

Their ultimate concern is the bottom line, but they understand that good staff morale is an investment that pays rather than a cost.

When people work for an organisation and a manager who they feel genuinely cares about their wellbeing and development they are likely to stay in their jobs for longer, take fewer days off sick and increase productivity and creativity.

development and happiness, they are more likely to stay in their job (reducing recruitment and HR costs), less likely to be off sick and more likely to work creatively and productively while they are in the building.

Ruthlessness isn't a prerequisite for success – benevolence and kindness can help attract a better calibre of employee.

Some of the most successful business people and civil servants have a strong history of philanthropy and excellent staff relations. Far from damaging their prospects, it has enhanced their reputation and helped them to recruit the best people to work with them.

Richard Branson is almost as well known for his positive image as his distinctive appearance.

Richard Branson, the founder and chairman of Virgin Group and the fourth richest person in Great Britain, enjoys an almost unilaterally positive image among the general public. This is unusual in a country where we are suspicious of those with money and the successful often fall victim to 'tall poppy syndrome'.

People who buy Virgin products are also buying into the Branson brand – as a distinctive leader (in his appearance as well as his personality) his name is synonymous with the business. He is a familiar figure on the world stage as a humanitarian committed to reducing environmental damage and Third World poverty and puts his money where his mouth is, making multi-million pound donations to good causes. The brand is now known within the healthcare sector

As a result people are generally happier to buy into a brand with someone such as this as its figurehead.

after he bought out a private medical company and set up Virgin Care, now a provider of NHS community services.

In the 1980s, a friend of mine complained about the rudeness of one of the staff in a Virgin Megastore and received a personal note from Branson apologising profusely for the incident. This happened nearly 30 years ago, and yet she still thinks favourably about the Virgin brand. You can't buy this kind of PR, because it comes from an individual who genuinely believes in making an effort to be personal and care about his customers as well as staff (Virgin always features in the 'best places to work' surveys as well).

A friend of mine once complained about the service they received in a Virgin Megastore. The result was a personal note from Richard Branson apologising for the incident. You can't buy this kind of PR.

Examples of people who are genuinely caring (and loved by their staff) include Sir John Sulston (a scientist who won a Nobel Prize in 2002), former Environment Secretary Hilary Benn, and even the man TV audiences love to hate – Simon Cowell. Each of these people treat their staff with care, generosity and kindness, resulting in well motivated, hard working teams who are committed to being as successful as possible.

Other notable examples of people who genuinely care for their staff include Sir John Sulston, Hilary Benn and even Simon Cowell.

Their attitude towards their staff fosters motivation, hard work and commitment in return.

Simon Cowell can also be used as a rather tongue-in-cheek example of another aspect of compassionate leadership – criticism. Cowell is well known for his scathing comments on television talent shows, and whilst I would not advocate this sort of performance feedback, it is vital to remember that *constructive* critical feedback is an occasionally overlooked aspect of compassionate leadership. Criticism that is focused on learning and not simply on chastisement shows employees that you can not only forgive mistakes but help them learn how to avoid them in the future, an action which has the double benefit of not only improving their performance but also strengthening their bond to an organisation; and a leader who wants to make their life better rather than just criticising them, something that might be great for TV ratings but not in real life.

Looking after your staff is a worthwhile exercise of course, but when you realise that your efforts extend beyond the personal to the professional, then it becomes a no-brainer. However, a fundamental aspect of this approach is to ensure that, whatever you do in regard to fostering staff wellbeing, it is done with authenticity and a genuine desire to look after the individuals who make your organisation tick. People are not stupid, they will be able to sniff out gimmicks and weak attempts at morale improvement, and this will have quite the opposite effect that you intend.

Constructive criticism is an important part of being a compassionate leader.

Ensure that you do criticise where necessary, but focus on the lessons learned and the future rather than just chastisement.

Ensure that whatever methods you adopt in looking after your staff are done with authenticity and a genuine desire to improve their lot.

Don't fall for cheap gimmicks to try and boost morale now and again – employees will sniff these out and your attempts will almost certainly backfire.

So how do you become a really great person to work with? The answer is "not overnight", but the following exercises will help you change the way you view your team which, in turn, will affect the way they behave both with you and their patients.

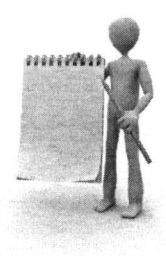

Exercises

Write down the names of people you admire who combine a strong work ethic and professional success with a kind, human side. Who would make your top five? In order to develop a more caring attitude in the workplace we need to be convinced that it is both desirable and possible. We *can* be successful and helpful/kind/generous, etc. We just need the evidence to make the case to ourselves.

In your notebook, write down the names of everyone you work with, including your line managers, and anyone who reports to you. Next to their name, write down what you consider to be their personal strengths and qualities. Are they kind? Helpful? Patient? Funny? It doesn't matter if it doesn't seem relevant to their role, just get it down on paper. Then jot down specific instances when they have displayed this behaviour. Did your manager stay late and talk to you about a personal problem you had? Did one of your team invite a new starter out for lunch because they seemed to be a bit lost? In the words of Oprah Winfrey, "what we focus on, expands". So it makes sense to focus on the good stuff.

Everyone has a strength, even if it appears to be outnumbered by weaknesses. The aim here is to concentrate on individual qualities. People will subconsciously respond better to someone who sees them as a kind person as opposed to a late person. It will improve your working relationships, and if you do this exercise with your spouse or partner it will improve your personal ones as well!

"Having a personality of caring about people is important. You can't be a good leader unless you generally like people. This is how you bring out the best in them."

Richard Branson

"If you want others to be happy, practice compassion. If you want to be happy, practice compassion."

Dalai Lama

"How far you go in life depends on your being tender with the young, compassionate with the aged, sympathetic with the striving and tolerant of the weak and strong. Because someday in your life you will have been all of these."

George Washington Carver

Chapter Three: Make it a habit

Most of us think about our habits in terms of the bad ones. Whether it's smoking, eating too many sausage rolls or watching reality TV, the association for many of us with the word 'habit' is to stop.

But the word is morally neutral – a habit is simply "a settled or regular tendency or practice" according to my dictionary. As Gandhi's quote at the end of this chapter implies, our habits, whether good or bad ones, affect the course of our lives, so it makes sense to consciously choose as many good ones as possible.

I will not be focusing on bad habits here, so if there are some that you would like to remove or replace, try to focus on the opposite, e.g. "eat more healthy foods" rather than "ditch the Mars bars". As we saw in the exercises of the last chapter, what we focus on increases so it makes sense to concentrate our energies and time on creating something positive, realistic and lasting.

There are many myths surrounding habits. One particularly common one is that it takes 21 repetitions of an activity to make it a habit. Or that you should only focus on changing one habit at a time. Both of these are untrue, and believing them may stand in your way of

The word 'habit' is often associated with something negative that should be stopped – how often do you hear the phrase 'good habit'?

However, the word 'habit' is morally neutral, but as they affect the course of our lives it makes sense to choose as many good ones as possible.

This book will not focus on bad habits, so try to think in terms of what you would like to gain rather than what you would like to quit – e.g. "eat healthier food" rather than "ditch the Mars bars".

You do not need to repeat something 21 times for it to become a habit.

Also, you don't need to concentrate on only changing one habit at a time.

taking action. You can create a habit in very little time if you know how to do it, and you can (and should) tackle several at once. The key to creating successful habits is to **keep them small**.

BJ Fogg, a social scientist and behavioural researcher at Stanford University, has developed a programme with an incredible success rate called Tiny Habits[2]. He believes that the reason we fail to maintain our desired habits (often formed in the guise of New Year's Resolutions) is because we are too ambitious, and that the distance from where we are now to where we want to be is too far.

As an example, he gives someone who wants to start jogging. Conventional wisdom would advise that person to go for a walk every day, then alternate jogging for a few minutes with walking, and eventually move on to continuous running. This may (and does) work for some people. But to improve your chances of success, his recommendation would be to simply put on a pair of trainers for the first five days. Do nothing else, but put on your shoes. After the next five days, you can move things forward, because your brain will already be totally comfortable with the unthreatening act of simply putting on a pair of shoes.

If approached in the right way you can create a habit in very little time.

Scientist and behavioural researcher BJ Fogg has developed a successful programme called Tiny Habits which involves managing unrealistic ambitions and focusing on small steps to a larger success.

To use the example of someone who wants to take up jogging, he argues that the first stage should be to simply put on a pair of trainers for five days, after which further smaller steps can be taken on the way to the larger task.

Fogg also recommends starting a new habit after an existing one. So if you are pretty confident in your habit of putting the kettle on for the first cup of tea in the office, this would be a good time to introduce the new one, such as eating a portion of fruit. He counsels against trying to introduce new habits in the middle of the day as it can be a chaotic time for many people. So by sticking to morning or night you are stacking the odds in your favour. In a professional setting, of course, this will mean the morning (unless you work night shifts).

How do you know which habits to adopt? In this book we are concerned with improving the care and compassion within your team (and wider organisation), so you might choose to think about your bigger goals. At the end of this chapter we will look at ways of transforming those overarching aims into concrete steps you can be confident of achieving.

At the end of the 1980s, a self-help book was published that took the business world by storm. It has sold more than 25 million copies, been translated into 38 languages and been praised by politicians worldwide (including Bill Clinton, who invited its author to Camp David to help him integrate the teachings of the book into his office).

Fogg recommends starting a new habit after an existing one, such eating a portion of fruit after making the morning cup of tea, thus tying the two actions together.

Fogg also recommends introducing new habits in the morning or evening rather than midway through a working day.

We are concerned with the field of healthcare, so consider your goals in this area.

In the late 1980s, a self-help book was written that took the business world by storm.

It has had many high profile proponents over the years, including Bill Clinton.

It is called *The 7 Habits of Highly Effective People*[3] by Stephen Covey, and is one of the most convincing texts on the need for interdependence in a leadership setting that I have encountered. The first three habits are concerned with the self, and include 'Be proactive', 'Begin with the end in mind' and 'Put first things first'. These are all very important, but it is the next three that have particular relevance for this book, so I will quote the summaries of each habit as well:

It is called 'The 7 Habits of Highly Effective People' and has sold over 25 million copies.

Habit 4: Think Win-Win
Genuinely strive for mutually beneficial solutions or agreements in your relationships. Value and respect people by understanding a 'win' for all is ultimately a better long-term resolution than if only one person in the situation had gotten his way.

Habit 4: Think Win-Win

Habit 5: Seek First to Understand, Then to be Understood
Use empathetic listening to be genuinely influenced by a person, which compels them to reciprocate the listening and take an open mind to being influenced by you. This creates an atmosphere of caring, and positive problem solving.

Habit 5: Seek First to Understand, Then to be Understood

Habit 6: Synergize

Combine the strengths of people through positive teamwork, so as to achieve goals no one person could have done alone.

If everyone working in healthcare were to observe these three habits, imagine what a change we would see! So many people pay lip service to the concept of teamwork, yet very few genuinely strive to achieve a 'win' for people other than themselves. Covey introduces the concept of the 'abundance mentality', where we can be reassured that there is enough for everyone, and that *my* success does not have to mean *your* failure.

He also coined the term 'scarcity mindset', where people close ranks and feel threatened by the success of others. This trait is particularly easy to slip into during a recession when resources are tight and savings have to come from somewhere. But operating from a position of scarcity stifles our creativity, keeps us attached to a 'them and us' mentality, and means we make our decisions from a place of fear rather than one of confidence and expansiveness.

I am not suggesting that you stick your head in the sand or pretend you have a larger budget or more staff than you really do, but I hope you can appreciate the

Habit 6: Synergize

The world of healthcare would be a very different place if those three habits were observed by those working within it!

Covey introduced the concept of the 'abundance mentality', where one success does not automatically mean a failure on the opposite side.

He also coined the term, 'scarcity mindset', where people close ranks and feel threatened by the success of others.

This trait is particularly easy to slip into during a recession. It stifles creativity and retains a 'them and us' mentality.

difference in mindset and that when it comes to communicating with and managing teams, adopting an attitude of kindness, generosity and patience will pay off far more handsomely than one of tension or competition.

This open and expansive approach will also inevitably benefit the most important person in the equation – the patient. Despite the motivation to help people that drives many who embark on a career in healthcare, it can be easy to lose sight of this as we climb the management ladder. Ultimately, all the goals, targets and KPIs that can fill our working hours are geared at improving care for the patient and meeting their needs as effectively and efficiently as possible. Developing habits that keep the patient as the main focus will have the win-win effect of optimising patient care as well as improving team focus and morale as everyone works towards a shared goal.

One of Stephen Covey's sons, also called Stephen, has followed in his father's footsteps and has identified an area he believes is becoming paramount in business – trust. Trust, Covey states, is the critical leadership competency of the modern economy, and it has a direct impact on costs and efficiency – as trust within an organisation increases, the speed at which things get

Adopting an attitude of kindness, generosity and patience will pay off far more handsomely than one of tension or competition.

It can be easy to lose the motivation that encouraged us to embark on a career in healthcare in the first place, but this more open approach ultimately helps the most important person in the equation – the patient.

All the goals, targets and KPIs that fill our working day are (or should be) geared towards helping patients. We should all aim to develop habits that optimise patient care.

Stephen Covey Jr advocates trust as the critical leadership competency of the modern economy.

done also increases and the cost required to do them goes down. The reverse, he claims, is also true – where little trust exists it takes longer to get things done, and therefore, it becomes more expensive as more checks are carried out at each stage. I'm sure almost all of you have experienced both ends of this scale during your time in a management position. The NHS is very different to other organisations in that its customers literally leave their lives in its employees' hands on a daily basis. Therefore, trust in the service provided is the single most important factor for patients, and is something that has its roots in the way that the multifarious sub-organisations and departments within the NHS, not to mention external contractors, deal with each other – something else that could be improved with a growth in trust.

On an individual level, trust in an employer and its leaders is a huge driver for an employee – they need to have faith that the leader they look up to is sure of their own abilities and aims. Covey makes a compelling business case for trust, and it is well worth your time investigating this area further.

An increase of trust within an organisation (and its external agencies) also increases the speed at which procedures are seen through whilst simultaneously reducing the cost.

Trust is particularly important for an organisation such as the NHS, where customers (patients) literally put their lives in the hands of the organisation.

The administrative side of the NHS, with all its sub-organisations, departments and contractors, requires trust to operate – trust that is not always present.

Individuals also need to have faith in their leader in order to follow them wholeheartedly and buy into their aims.

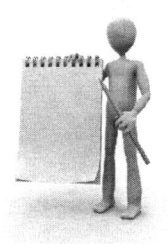

Exercises

Pick three goals you'd like to achieve regarding care and compassion in your workplace. Looking at your list of areas to work on that you made in Chapter One should give you some good ideas.

Let's use as an example:

1. Develop a stronger team spirit
2. Keep the patient and their needs as the number one priority
3. Make the working environment a more enjoyable place to be

Break this down into smaller chunks. These might be:

1. Go for lunches or after work drinks together.
2. Make a point of asking each staff member about their patients

3. Hold a meeting about physical improvements that can be made to the workplace.

The micro habits that come from this could therefore be:

1. Write down the name of one staff member each day on a piece of paper entitled, "team lunch"

2. At the top of your to-do list each morning, write the word "patient care" so that it informs everything listed below

3. Write down a simple and brief suggestion for improving things in your notebook every morning

The key is to do this every day for five days. It might seem a bit ludicrous to start the process of getting people together by simply writing their name down, but it will get the ball rolling mentally. It will also keep you subconsciously on the alert for possible ideas – you may find things start to happen without you actively doing anything!

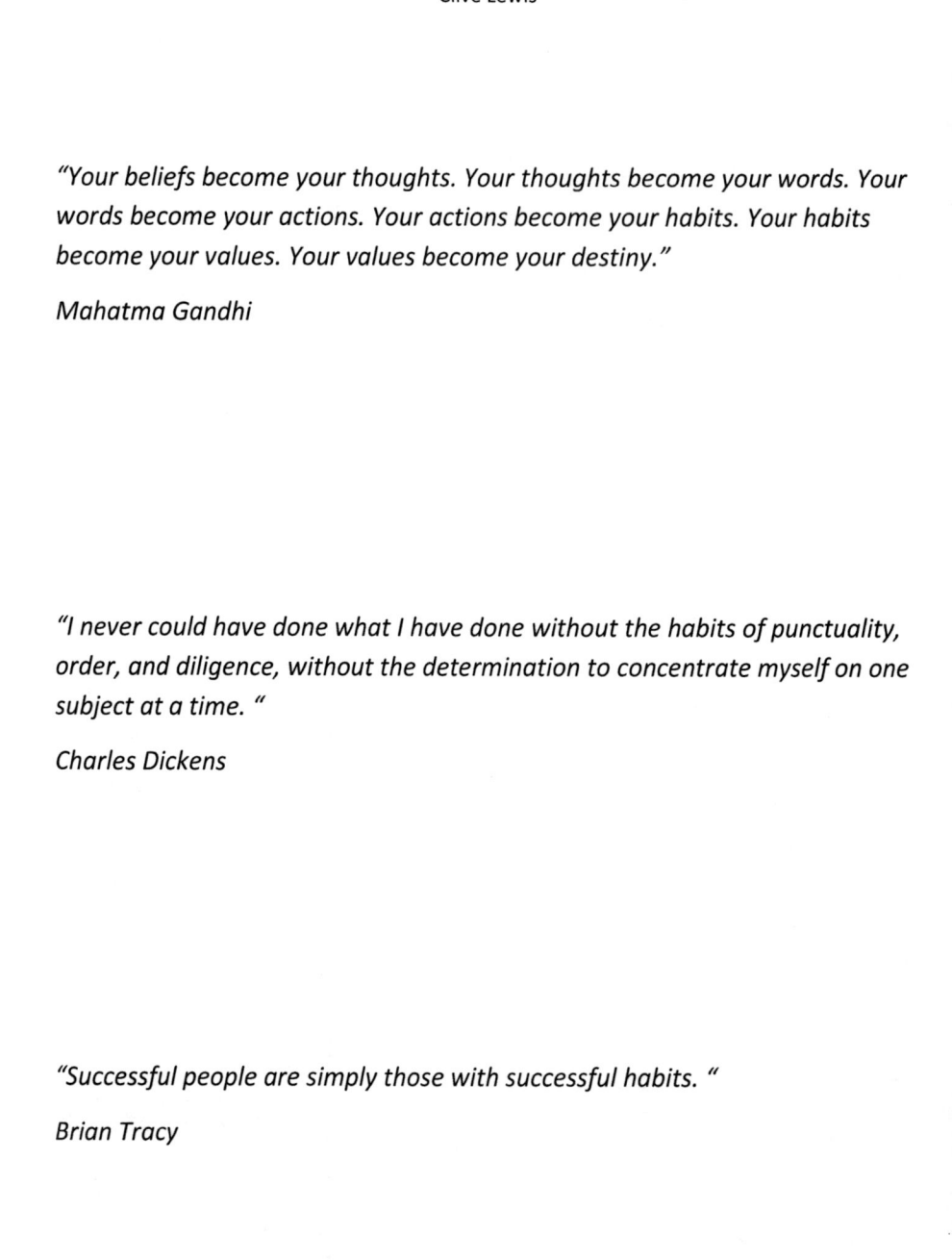

"Your beliefs become your thoughts. Your thoughts become your words. Your words become your actions. Your actions become your habits. Your habits become your values. Your values become your destiny."

Mahatma Gandhi

"I never could have done what I have done without the habits of punctuality, order, and diligence, without the determination to concentrate myself on one subject at a time. "

Charles Dickens

"Successful people are simply those with successful habits. "

Brian Tracy

Chapter Four: Be inspired

As we saw in Chapter Two, it is very important to have role models to whom we can look for inspiration in our quest to be more compassionate leaders. I hope that you are already channelling your inner Richard Branson or John Sulston, or whoever you selected as your hero in the field!

Role models are important when it comes to finding inspiration for our transition to more compassionate leaders.

However, it is also beneficial to be motivated by real life figures who can keep your energy and enthusiasm high when life gets in the way. We may have already integrated certain positive habits (tiny or otherwise) into our working day, but for the big picture and a sense of vision, nothing beats having a mentor.

A real life figure can also act as an inspiration. To this end, nothing beats having a mentor.

Mentoring used to be considered a bit "alternative" in many businesses, but today it is absolutely mainstream and many large organisations will already have an established mentoring programme for their managers. But what exactly is mentoring? And how can it help you come closer to achieving your goals?

Mentoring has gone from being an unusual method of employee development to being much more mainstream across the business spectrum.

What is mentoring?

In brief, mentoring is all about helping someone achieve a goal or situation that is important to them, in a supportive and kindly way. Mentors may come from any

In brief, mentoring is all about helping someone achieve a goal or situation that is important to them, in a supportive and kindly way.

field and do not have to be directly related to your own sphere of experience; however, it can be helpful if they have a broad appreciation of your concerns and the sector in which you work. It is also recommended that your mentor is not your line manager or anyone connected to your organisation. This way the advice they give can remain impartial, and will not be affected by anything you disclose about your activities or working relationships.

Mentors shouldn't be your line manager or someone connected to your organisation.

It is important that mentors are impartial and not affected by any of your activities or working relationships.

To put coaching and mentoring into an official context, the EMCC (European Mentoring and Coaching Council), the body to which the NHS adheres in its coaching and mentoring standards, offers the following definitions[4]:

Coaching: "Coaching is facilitating the client's learning process by using professional methods and techniques to help the client to improve what is obstructive and nurture what is effective, in order to reach the client's goals."

Mentoring: "Mentoring can be described as a developmental process which may involve a transfer of skill or knowledge from a more experienced to a less experienced person through learning dialogue and role modelling, and may also be a learning partnership between peers."

How does it work?

Most mentoring sessions take place offsite in a neutral setting to underline the impartiality of the relationship but also to help you think, quite literally, 'outside the box'. The format of the sessions will be agreed in advance – some people prefer a structured conversation and to report on the progress of activities since the last session, while others like to take a more general, "what's going on with me right now" approach. It is helpful to consider your favoured style when selecting a mentor, as it is important that you develop a strong rapport for the mentoring relationship to be a success.

Mentoring sessions usually take place offsite to reinforce the impartiality of the relationship.

Session formats will usually be agreed in advance but can take many forms, from structured conversations to practical exercises.

If you choose a more relaxed approach, try not to stray into therapeutic territory. Your mentor may be very open and easy to talk to, but their role is to advise you in a professional sense. By all means discuss your feelings about work, but keep it focused. If you find that more personal issues arise from your discussions, seek out a counsellor and see them in a different capacity.

Don't forget that your mentor is not your therapist – you are both there in a professional context.

How will it help me?

The Institute of Healthcare Management[5] identifies the following benefits to the mentee:

- Fundamental shifts in personal skills and self-awareness

- The development of a lifelong approach to self-directed learning

- Enhanced acquisition of managerial competence

- The development of networks across a broader spectrum than that provided by the normal environment

- Enhanced capacity to make sense of and apply learning within the organisational context

- Enhanced ability to source new ideas and practices from outside the organisation and integrate them into it

- Enhanced self-awareness, autonomy and self-confidence

Too good to be true? Not really. As a mentee you receive the benefits mentioned above and pass them on to your team and the wider organisation. It doesn't have to take a lot of time (you can choose to meet once a week, once a fortnight or once a month, whatever your calendars will allow), so even the strictest of line managers should be open to the idea.

As a mentee, you will benefit personally from what you have learned, but your team will also benefit when you put your new learnings into practice.

How do I choose a mentor?

If you work in the NHS, your Trust may already have an established mentoring programme, but if yours doesn't, or you work in private healthcare, you may need to forge your own path. Consider the following:

Your Trust may already have a mentoring programme established, but you can do it yourself if they don't.

- Ask your HR department. Even if there is no formal programme in place, other managers in your organisation may be being mentored

- Use your networks, whether online (such as LinkedIn) or real life gatherings. Talk to people and let them know you're looking for a mentor. There is no stigma attached, and people are often pleased to be asked (both for recommendations, and to be a mentor)

- Look back over your CV. Maybe an old boss or colleague in a former organisation would be a good candidate

- If you're a member of a professional association or trade union, they may be able to help

- Have realistic expectations of what they can do. You can't expect a mentor to make decisions for you or make changes on your behalf. Their role is advisory and motivational

- Don't be disheartened if your prospective mentor declines your invitation. Most people are very flattered to be asked, but may not be able to spare the time. Dust yourself down and move onto your next choice

Have your own vision

Spending time with an inspirational leader can give you the impetus to help others in turn. Although it would be inappropriate for you to formally mentor members of your team, you do want to project your enthusiasm and passion for care. For your team to benefit from this you need to have a vision for your team/department's work. It needs to be uplifting and make you feel excited and optimistic when you read/say it out loud. You don't need to share it if you choose not to, but write it down in your notebook. If you're stuck for inspiration, have a look at your organisation's corporate vision, or that of a company you admire. Almost everyone includes this on their website these days.

Your experiences with mentoring may in turn give you the impetus to help others.

You should have an uplifting vision for your team/department's work.

The key to getting other people to share your sense of purpose is to help them achieve their own goals. It may sound counterintuitive, but you need to put yourself in their shoes and identify their priorities. What really matters to them? Self-interest is not always a negative –

Helping other people achieve their own goals is key to getting others to share your enthusiasm.

it is what motivates most of us in our daily lives. There will be some part of your vision that chimes with each member of your team, but it might be different for each person. For one person, making the patient feel valued and respected may be their priority. For another, even though they also care about this, they may be more motivated by external praise from a department head, or the satisfaction of a completed project. Identify the payoffs to each of your team, and they will follow you. As business coach and mentor Fiona Harrold[6] suggests, tell yourself "I will succeed in my objectives in helping others achieve theirs".

Identifying what motivates your team and the individuals within it can be difficult work, but it is rewarding and will take you well on the way towards your goal of being a compassionate leader.

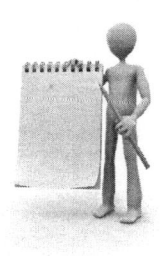

Exercises

If the idea of mentoring appeals to you, have a conversation with your line manager about it. Sell them the benefits to your organisation and team. The time you invest will be repaid many times over.

Spend some time researching possible mentors. There are a lot of good resources out there that offer templates for mentoring agreements and information on what to expect (and how to cope if, for any reason, the mentoring relationship should break down). Just Google "mentoring in the NHS" and you will find a wealth of information. There are some other suggested links in the reference section at the back of the book[7-8].

Whether you choose to be mentored or not, don't forget to inspire your own team. You don't have to ask them directly about what matters to them – it will become clear as you get to know them better. Jot down in your notebook what you think their priorities are, and drop them into conversation when discussing your vision. You may be surprised by how effective this is!

"Advice is like snow; the softer it falls, the longer it dwells upon, and the deeper it sinks into the mind."

Samuel Taylor Coleridge

"Mentoring is a brain to pick, an ear to listen, and a push in the right direction."

John Crosby

"I've learned that people will forget what you said, people will forget what you did, but people will never forget how you made them feel."

Maya Angelou

Chapter Five - Take time out

What are you feeling right now? How about your body, are there any aches or pains? How are you breathing? What's going through your mind?

Most of us have to stop and think for a while about these questions as we can so easily be detached from our own bodily experience. This is especially true when we're at work and may be dealing with several people and situations at once.

If we were asked, most of us would have to stop and actually think about how we really feel, especially in a stressful work environment.

The problem with operating on autopilot is that we may react to circumstances without really thinking it through. When we spend all day on high alert we can feel stressed and out of control, which in turn affects the dynamic within our team. It is also difficult to keep our priorities in mind when we have lots of deadlines and feel that everyone 'wants a piece of us' – we tend to respond to the other person's sense of urgency, rather than what *we've* decided is important.

Operating on autopilot means that we can sometimes react to circumstances without actually thinking them through.

One strategy for dealing with this habit of overreacting is to integrate mindfulness practice and techniques into daily life. Mindfulness has become something of a buzzword within the healthcare profession in recent times, but its efficacy in reducing stress is well documented.

'Mindfulness' has become something of a buzzword within the healthcare profession in recent times, but its efficacy in reducing stress is well documented.

Although service users typically benefit from mindfulness programmes (such as those receiving treatment for depression, OCD or chronic pain), there are now a number of courses aimed at healthcare practitioners themselves. A recent report in the Journal of the American Medical Association[9] looked at whether mindfulness could help primary care physicians improve their own wellbeing and capacity to relate to patients and reduce burnout and stress. The study reported "...sustained improvements in well-being and attitudes associated with patient centred care. Staff experienced improved personal well-being, increased empathy and psychosocial beliefs and a reduction in feelings of emotional exhaustion, and depersonalization."

Another study of 27 healthcare professionals at McGill University in Montreal[10] found "participants had enhanced awareness of and ability to disengage from ruminative thoughts, and they reported increases in self-care practices and psychological well-being after the course". It may be something of a cliché, but these studies demonstrate that looking after ourselves means we can provide better care for others.

A recent report in the Journal of the American Medical Association found that practising mindfulness reduced stress, emotional exhaustion and depersonalisation in the healthcare sector and improved attitudes associated with patient centred care.

A study at McGill University in Montreal found that practising mindfulness increased participant "awareness of and ability to disengage from ruminative thoughts."

The study also reported increases in psychological wellbeing of the participants.

Looking after ourselves therefore clearly improves our ability to better care for others.

What is mindfulness?

Jon Kabat-Zinn, a renowned teacher of mindfulness meditation and founder of the Mindfulness-Based Stress Reduction programme at the University of Massachusetts, defines mindfulness as, "paying attention in a particular way; on purpose, in the present moment, and nonjudgmentally."[11]

In practice, this means focusing on the experience you are having, as you are having it. So, if you are holding this book, you become aware of how your fingers feel on the page, the way your back and rest of your body feel as you are sitting down, how you are holding your head, the way you are breathing, the thoughts and feelings you are having as you read the words, etc. If this seems a lot to take in at once – it is. Most mindfulness programmes start small, with a focus on the way the breath feels as you inhale and exhale, and on the bodily sensations you experience as you breathe.

One of the main cornerstones of mindfulness meditation is regular practice. Every programme requires you to commit some time on a daily basis, but its benefits in your professional and personal life can be significant.

Mindfulness guru Jon Kabat-Zinn defines mindfulness as: "paying attention in a particular way; on purpose, in the present moment, and nonjudgmentally."

In practice, this means focusing on the experience you are having, as you are having it.

Be aware of what you are touching, hearing and smelling, how it feels and how it makes you feel.

It may be too much to take in at first, but most mindfulness programmes start small for this very reason and build up.

Regular, daily practice is the key to advancing in mindfulness.

Professor Michael West of Lancaster University Management School[12] cites the following as why mindfulness is important for leadership:

- Being present in interactions
- Knowing one's own motivations, moods and feelings
- Choosing positive emotions (supportive rather than resentful)
- Observing our own reactions and creating space
- Being aware of the needs of others
- Managing meetings
- Maintaining a focus on priorities
- Value driven behaviour – mindfulness as a route to the fundamental
- Leadership is being mindful of people and tasks

It may seem something of a leap to go from focusing on how our neck feels to managing our meetings better or improving patient care, but the two are connected. Every time we become conscious of our body and fully inhabit it, we feel more grounded. When you are aware of being present in the moment, you are less likely to be affected by feelings of how you have reacted in the

Every time we become conscious of our body and fully inhabit it, we feel more grounded.

past, and more able to choose your response to the situation. When we are in a state of reaction and 'out of body-ness', our response can sometimes be triggered by the memory of a past experience. Being aware of and in control of our thoughts means we are in a better position to choose a more helpful response. This is particularly important when working in healthcare, as decisions that we take in haste can have significant repercussions for frontline workers, and therefore for patients.

Our present feelings will eventually replace our past reactions to events.

There are already a number of mindfulness programmes available for workers in some NHS Trusts such as the Black Country Partnership, Lancashire Care and Nottinghamshire Healthcare, and those who run such programmes may offer similar courses for private healthcare agencies. You may also like to investigate some of these dedicated programmes for your staff (depending on training budgets). To appreciate the personal benefits of mindfulness, try to practise some of the simple techniques suggested below every day.

An increase in mindfulness would also boost another area the NHS is looking to improve in its staff – resilience. Increasing staff resilience, that is the ability to deal effectively and swiftly with stressful/changeable situations, would not only be of benefit to the individual

Increasing resilience improves performance and efficiency and drives down sickness and related costs, as well as benefitting the individual themselves.

members of staff themselves but would also increase performance and efficiency across whole departments, whilst simultaneously driving down sickness and the related costs to the service. Resilience is a term that will almost certainly become more prevalent in NHS lexicon over the next few years, but those who wish to get ahead of the game might like to undertake the free Robertson Cooper i-resilience report[13] to test their own current resilience levels and see how an increase in resilience could benefit them and their department.

Resilience is set to become a prominent area of NHS focus in the coming years.

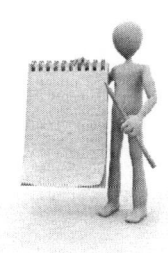

Exercises

Everyday actions. Pick something you do every day, such as washing your face or brushing your teeth, and really concentrate on the experience. How does your arm and shoulder feel as you lift it to your face? What does the toothpaste smell like? How does the water feel on your face? Try and notice as many things as you can about your body and the sensations you're experiencing.

Breath awareness. Set a timer for five minutes, sit up straight, and become aware of your breath going in and out. Notice how it feels going in through your nostrils, how it feels as it travels through your body to your chest or stomach, and how it feels again on the exhale. Every time your mind wanders (and it will do, as that's what minds do) come back to the feeling of the breath in your body. Try and do this every day, and gradually extend the time you spend on your practice.

Mindful movement. Next time you have to walk any distance, try and concentrate on the whole motion of the heel, then the rest of the foot coming into contact with the ground. Notice how the back, hips, shoulders and neck feel. You can do this if you do any other type of exercise, such as swimming or yoga. Keep bringing the awareness back to your physical sensations every time the mind gets lost in fantasy or daydream.

Integrate mindfulness into your working life. When you arrive at your desk, really feel your body sit down in the chair and become aware of the space you take up. Before a meeting, take a few moments to focus on the breath, even if you have to nip to the toilets to get a bit of privacy! A meeting where you feel calm and present will be much more productive for all parties.

If you are drawn to studying the techniques you are learning in greater depth, there are many books, DVDs and courses (distance learning, online and face to face) available[14].

Even if you feel sceptical, give these exercises a try for a week or so. You won't have wasted much time if you decide they're not for you, and you might discover some techniques that can benefit you personally, as well as your wider team.

"Suffering usually relates to wanting things to be different from the way they are."

Allan Lokos

"Respond; don't react. Listen; don't talk. Think; don't assume."

Raji Lukkoor

"Mindfulness is simply being aware of what is happening right now without wishing it were different; enjoying the pleasant without holding on when it changes (which it will); being with the unpleasant without fearing it will always be this way (which it won't)."

James Baraz

Chapter Six - Get a fresh perspective

One of the reasons people enter the healthcare profession is because they want to help others. Despite this, many of us are determined to do things 'our own way'. This is natural – we see our environment through the prism of our background, learning and experience, and may have a strong sense about how the world 'should' be.

Problems can arise, however, when our view of something clashes with someone else's. They may be a team member, our manager or a member of the public. When we get stuck in conflict about who is right about a particular idea or decision we lose our opportunity to demonstrate empathy and compassion. Nothing says "I care" less than a dogmatic, inflexible stance.

One thing the best managers and leaders all have in common is their ability to quickly establish rapport with their interlocutor. Have you ever met someone who instantly made you feel more confident, at ease, and that they really cared about what you had to say? Either consciously or unconsciously, they were building rapport with you. And people like people who make them feel good. They become more productive, more creative, and more enjoyable to spend time with. So

It is natural as we progress through our careers that our experiences shape the way we view our environment.

Problems arise however when our views clash with the views of others.

We can become locked in a conflict which goes against our aim of being a compassionate, empathetic individual.

Most of us have met someone who instantly made us feel more confident and at ease, and appeared to really care about what we had to say.

This is called building rapport.

how can you create a strong rapport with anyone you meet? By adopting some easy techniques borrowed from the Neuro-Linguistic Programming (NLP) approach to personal development we can improve relationships with colleagues and patients overnight. NLP is a personal development programme used by individuals, businesses and governments that utilises a perceived connection between the neurological processes, language and behavioural patterns learned through experience that can be changed to achieve specific goals.

Rapport building is key to becoming a compassionate leader.

Neuro-Linguistic Programming (NLP) features long standing techniques for rapport building.

Creating rapport by 'matching'

Try this little experiment with a friend or colleague when you've got some time and there's nothing important at stake. While you're talking, try to mirror their physical position and movement. If they've got their legs crossed, cross yours too. If their head is slightly tilted to one side, do the same. Be subtle though, there's no need to turn into Marcel Marceau.

Now notice how they're speaking and try to match the speed and tone of your voice to theirs. If they have a naturally deep voice, lower yours a notch too. We all have a broad vocal spectrum so it's possible to change

Matching involves subtly mirroring your interlocutor in tone, actions and manner.

yours a little without sounding unnatural or as if you're doing an impersonation.

Notice how you feel. Do you find the conversation flows more easily? Are you able to find common ground?

You will often find that the conversation flows more easily and you can find common ground.

Now make a conscious move to mismatch. Tune your voice to a shade higher or lower than theirs. Talk more quickly or slowly than they do (whichever will be less obvious). Change your posture. What do you notice? It's likely that the train of your conversation will abruptly change and maybe even stop. Mismatching is the antithesis of what you should do to create rapport, but it's a great technique to use when you want to end a conversation quickly!

Purposefully mismatching will demonstrate the power of matching – the conversation will likely stutter and stop or at least be very awkward.

You can also mirror with language. It can be tempting to paraphrase someone when we want to show we've understood their point, but it's actually more effective to use their own words (not totally verbatim, of course, you want to make someone feel you're speaking their language, not sounding like a parrot.) So if they talk about feeling blue, don't leap to label them as 'depressed' in the next sentence. Using people's original language is reassuring for them, and you may actually discover that they meant something a little different from your interpretation of the term.

You can also mirror with language.

Using a selection of the words someone says to you in your responses can be an easy way of showing that you have understood the other person's point.

Once you've played around with matching and mismatching in informal situations, you can use it during meetings, one to ones and other times when you want to establish rapport. Subtly change your body language (and verbal language) to match theirs. You will soon feel more in tune with one another, leading to better and more productive encounters and working relationships.

Pacing and leading

Imagine you are facing a patient who is angry that his operation has been postponed. His life has been significantly inconvenienced by this news, he may be in pain for longer and he may have to change the time he had booked off work. His voice is loud, he is making big gestures with his arms and speaking in a fast and agitated manner.

If you start to engage with him in a soft, slow voice, he will probably interpret it as patronising. Your calm is just further evidence to him that you're not affected and that you don't care. In creating this disconnect you are unlikely to reach an easy truce. You're immediately pitting yourself against him, even though it's instinctive to use a calm tone in an attempt to diffuse the situation.

Once you have experimented with matching in informal situations, try taking it into a business scenario.

Pacing and leading involves matching (or nearly matching) your opposite number before slowly drawing them away from their stance to where you would like them to be in order to achieve your goal.

Imagine you are facing a patient who is angry that his operation has been cancelled. His voice is loud, he is making big gestures with his arms and speaking in a fast and agitated manner.

It may appear natural to try and calm him down, but he may take your calm voice as evidence that you are unaffected by the news.

It may appear counterintuitive, but it can help if you increase the speed and volume of your voice and movements to nearly match his (if he's really shouting, don't aim for exactly the same level or you'll end up in a slanging match!). This is 'pacing'. You need to try and get onto his wavelength in order to then slightly lower your voice and slow down your movements. Do this gradually, and you will probably find that he will too. This is known as 'leading'. You are far more likely to get cooperation and understanding from another person when they feel that you 'get them'. Of course, the content is up to you – unfortunately good communication will not solve the problem of the delayed operation in the first place!

Try increasing the volume of your voice and the speed of your speech before slightly bringing both down to a more tolerable level.

You will likely find that he will mirror your pattern. This is pacing.

Multiple description

This is a rather technical-sounding term for "seeing things from another perspective", but it is a good technique for appreciating differing points of view. Essentially, there are three 'positions' in an exchange between two people:

- First position – your own perception of what happened
- Second position – the other person's point of view

Multiple description simply means "seeing things from another perspective".

- Third position — how a detached observer may see the situation

If you're experiencing conflict with a team member or manager, using this technique can help you appreciate their take on the issue without losing sight of your own opinions or reality. First, think about the matter from your point of view. How do you feel? Why? What, in your opinion, should be done? Now, get up, have a little walk about, then sit down again and imagine you are the other person. What are they thinking and feeling? What is their point? Why have they taken the path they have? Again, stand up and stop your train of thought. Now, put yourself into 'third position'. What, in your view, is happening to the two parties? Where can you see the conflict? Seeing them express their feelings as they do, can you see any common ground or possible solution? Sometimes literally stepping outside your own head can help you find a more creative solution to a problem.

Utilising this technique in a situation of conflict can help you see another's viewpoint without losing sight of your own.

First, consider the matter from your own point of view.

Next, think of the same event from the other party's point of view.

Finally, how would an external person view the situation?

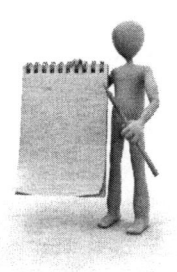

Exercises

Practise matching and mismatching with some friends and family. Become comfortable with altering your voice and body according to the person you're with. Make sure you consciously return to 'yourself' afterwards, though! Spending too long matching someone who is feeling miserable, for example, can leave you feeling bad unless you actively step out of the state.

When you feel happy matching in situations of little consequence, try the technique in more formal situations, such as a meeting. Write down anything you notice about the quality of your interactions after you have consciously mirrored the person you're with.

When pacing and leading it's very important to feel comfortable with the technique. Again, practise in your everyday life before bringing it into the work environment.

If you find these techniques useful you may like to investigate ways of formally introducing it into your work. There are plenty of NLP trainers who are experienced working in healthcare environments[15].

"If there is any one secret of success, it lies in the ability to get the other person's point of view and see things from that person's angle as well as from your own."

Henry Ford

"When you really listen to another person from their point of view, and reflect back to them that understanding, it's like giving them emotional oxygen."

Stephen Covey

"We cling to our own point of view, as though everything depended on it. Yet our opinions have no permanence; like autumn and winter, they gradually pass away."

Zhuangzi

Clive Lewis

Chapter Seven: Keeping it real

We live in a world where technology permeates every second of our waking life. Smartphones have made emails and social media ever more accessible, and our work lives are highly computer-led. How many times have you sent an email or instant message to someone in the same room? Digital technology has made many things more efficient (such as computerised patient records enabling clinicians to cross reference databases) but there is no evidence that our lives are any less stressful as a result. Indeed, the pressure to instantly respond to an email or Tweet can create anxiety and an expectation of expedience that simply didn't exist two decades ago.

Digital technology has made many things more efficient, but there is no evidence to suggest that it has made life less stressful.

It's ironic then that, while we have made significant and impressive advances in technology, 90% of what we communicate remains non-verbal. There are so many opportunities for misunderstandings with a written message, and the brevity that is now expected of our communications means the tone (and often the content) can be misconstrued. It's no coincidence that as more people choose to interact online rather than in person or on the phone, the number of 'smileys' and exclamation marks in our written communication has increased. It's as if we are desperate to reach through the computer

Despite the advances in technology, 90% of what we communicate remains non-verbal.

Misunderstanding is a natural consequence of a growth in written communication – for example, tone of voice is almost impossible to read in an email or a text.

screen and show the other person that we are a human being with feelings.

Marissa Mayer, the chief executive of Yahoo!, made the headlines for refusing to allow staff to work 100% remotely. For although the technological capabilities exist thanks to video conferencing, Skype etc., being able to see another person on a screen is not enough. No one has ever successfully led a team or an organisation from behind a computer. Ms Mayer came under fire for the new 'family-unfriendly' policy as many people had got used to working from home. Incidentally, she didn't say staff could never work from home, rather, that full-time remote working didn't foster a good team spirit. She acknowledged that flexible working is important, and staff need to feel valued. But for an organisation to have a sense of coherence and unity, its people need to be physically in the same place at least some of the time.

I'm not suggesting that you go ahead and cancel your team's work-from-home requests – that would *not* be appropriate in a book about care and compassion. It's also highly unrealistic for ward-based frontline care staff anyway! It's wonderful that technology has enabled us to connect virtually, and it is a useful tool when used wisely. I'm just saying that it's important to check in

Marissa Mayer, the chief executive of Yahoo!, announced to staff that 100% remote working was to end.

Whilst her policy wasn't well received, its intentions were clear – she believed that full-time remote working was bad for team spirit.

Whilst we should embrace technology in many situations, using it as a substitute for physical interaction isn't recommended.

with the whites of your co-workers' eyes on a regular basis.

We also need unscheduled face to face communication, even at work. In addition to formal meetings, the contact we have at the vending machine or in the lift is incredibly important, especially for managers. How else do you really know how your team is working? How can you know what is going on beneath the veneer of "fine" and "busy, busy" unless you have an opportunity to see them out of the formal manager/employee context?

Unscheduled face to face meetings, such as catching someone in the lift or on their way into the office, can help you get a feel for how your staff really are.

Have a think back to your communications today. Roughly what percentage would you say were conducted online and how many were face to face? Don't spend too long worrying about accuracy, but the chances are you'll have fired off 50 - 100 emails during the course of the day if you're largely deskbound. Then think about the face to face communications you had. What are the outcomes that you remember from the different types of communication? Of course, if you had some major news delivered via email, you're going to remember that. But we do tend to remember the conversations we had in person, followed by those over the phone, and last of all the emails.

Compare the communication methods you have used today – what percentage were face to face and what percentage were electronic?

From which of those encounters do you remember the outcomes? The chances are you remember more from an average face to face encounter than an electronic one.

I'm not suggesting that we do away with emails altogether – for a start it would be hugely impractical, and it's especially important in a healthcare organisation to have a paper trail (or its electronic equivalent) documenting actions taken, decisions made, etc. But I suspect there are a few areas where you could increase the human element of communication. Are you copying people into emails out of habit when you could go and speak to them? People easily get information overload. Ask yourself with every email, "do I need to send this? Does this person need this information in this way?" Often the answer will be "yes, because it's much quicker and I can't waste time with small talk when an information transfer is sufficient". That's fine, and demonstrates technology being used as it should. But where there are opportunities for personal interaction and they are the most appropriate medium for the message, use them. It may feel a little strange, especially if you have been used to putting everything in writing, but your team (and your managers) will appreciate it.

With patient contact the personal touch is hugely important, but can also be very challenging. People usually only come to you when there is something the matter with themselves or a loved one, and may feel frightened, angry, and more sensitive than usual. It is tempting in these situations to retreat behind computer

We shouldn't disregard electronic communication of course, but human interaction should make up a percentage of your daily communications – especially in a leadership scenario.

With your next communication, consider whether your intended medium is the most effective or whether a personal visit or phone call would be more beneficial. Leaders should be seen as well as heard.

In healthcare, your only contact with patients will usually only be when something is wrong with themselves or a loved one.

screens and official jargon, as they may seem to offer a temporary shield between ourselves and the other person's strong emotions. But people feel respected when they are looked in the eye and genuinely listened to. Everyone wants to be heard, and it makes our jobs much more rewarding when we can do this for people, however difficult the encounter might be.

It can be tempting to use a screen or even a phone as a shield, but ultimate patient respect lies in the personal touch – someone to look them in the eye and listen without barriers.

This is something that all of the role models we saw in Chapter Two have in common – they are all 'in person' people. All the bosses in the top 100 companies to work for spend a lot of face time with their employees, according to those who voted for them. Good leaders spend time on the 'shop floor', whether that is a factory or a hospital. Even if your job is not customer facing it's important to spend some time with the people you are ultimately there to help. You will be more responsive to their needs, spot problems quicker, and be an ambassador for care in your organisation. No one, regardless of their seniority, should be above talking to the people they are there to serve.

All of the role models discussed in Chapter Two are 'in person' people, as are all the bosses in the top 100 companies, according to their staff.

Good leaders spend time on the 'shop floor'. Although this isn't always possible in a leadership role, it's important to find a way of regularly speaking as directly as possible to those who use your service.

If you feel uncertain or fearful about communicating with people directly, we will look at ways to increase your confidence and sense of self-esteem in the next chapter.

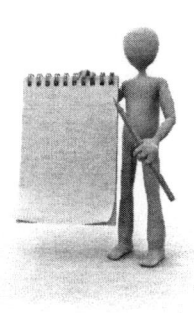

Exercises

Write down in your notebook what is preventing you from engaging in face to face communication. Is it fear of others? Worries about wasting time? Are you simply out of the habit? How can you address this? Is it a case of getting out of your comfort zone and doing it anyway? Or are there organisational issues you need to address? Face to face communication with co-workers and patients is really important, so change whatever is necessary to maximise your time.

Check your habits. Are you cc-ing people into emails to cover your back? Because you feel it somehow enhances your status? Do you really need to send this email or could it be added as a point in your next meeting or one to one? We have so much information to take in at work, so make sure you're part of the solution, not the problem.

"Face-to-face communication remains the most powerful human interaction."

Kathleen Begley

"Consistent, daily face-to-face communication promotes more than just good feelings; it also promotes effective and collaborative teamwork."

Gary McClain and Deborah Romaine

"Everybody gets so much information all day long that they lose their common sense."

Gertrude Stein

Chapter Eight: Respect begins at home

"What is a chapter about self-esteem doing in a book about leadership in healthcare?" you might be wondering. "I want to learn about instilling a culture of care and compassion in my organisation, not asking myself whether I was praised as a child".

The quote from Confucius at the end of this section says it all. Without a healthy dose of self-esteem, it is difficult to be a strong and caring leader. All the best bosses (those who lead by inspiration and enthusiasm rather than fear) feel good about themselves and their mission. Self-respect oozes from their every pore.

A strong, caring leader needs a healthy dose of self-esteem. The best bosses feel good about themselves and their mission.

The foundations to our self-esteem are laid very early in life. As children, we tend to take everything that is said to us at face value, and if the messages we receive are negative or demeaning, it will affect our self-image as adults. Chances are that if I asked you to list some of your weaknesses, many of them would have been internalised from things people told you as a child.

Our childhoods have a huge impact on our self-esteem and self-image.

As children we take what we are told at face value and usually carry this through to adulthood.

How does low self-esteem affect us in the workplace?

1. Perfectionism. Those who don't value themselves need to make sure everything is 'right', at whatever cost. If you have perfectionist

tendencies, you may suffer from anxiety and stress because there are so many things out of your control. It is hard to be managed by a perfectionist boss – you may be intolerant of human weaknesses in your team, who find it difficult to tell you when mistakes have been made

Perfectionism often breeds feelings of a lack of control and desperation to make sure that everything is 'right' at whatever cost.

2. Being critical of ourselves and others. Those who suffer from low self-esteem judge themselves harshly. Their self talk can be very negative, focusing on what is wrong in a situation to the exclusion of anything positive. An overly critical boss will sap team morale and contribute to high staff turnover

Those with low self-esteem are often super critical of themselves and others, often focusing on what is wrong and not what is right.

3. Fear of change. When life is predictable we experience the illusion of control, which helps us to feel safe. Feeling safe is very important for those with low self-esteem, but it can also stifle change and creativity. Along with change comes the risk of failure as well as the possibility of improvement. Bad practice can lay undetected for years because "things have always been done this way"

Feeling safe is very important to those with low self-esteem, stifling new thinking and creativity.

4. Addictions. Very prevalent within the healthcare sector as a coping mechanism, dependency on

Addictions are often used as a coping mechanism

alcohol, drugs, overeating, overspending and work are all symptoms of poor self-image

5. Being a victim. Do you struggle to say no to something or someone, then complain about how badly you've been treated? Do you take on more work than you should and become ill as a result? Lack of assertiveness and fear of other people's reactions is another indicator of low self-esteem

Those with low self-esteem struggle to say no to people, despite the potential cost to themselves or the inability to carry out the task.

Do you recognise yourself in any of these descriptions? Don't worry if you do – most people suffer from poor self-image from time to time. However, if you feel that low self-esteem is seriously affecting your life and wellbeing, please go to see a professional therapist or counsellor for help.

Many of us suffer from poor self-image from time to time, although large-scale or debilitating feelings of this nature should be tackled through professional help.

Actions that enhance your self-esteem

1. Setting and achieving goals. Deciding what you want in your personal and work life and taking steps to achieve it can really boost your self-esteem. They provide the evidence that you are capable and successful in your activity of choice. The key is to identify short and long-term goals. If your intention is to be CEO of your organisation, you will need to break down all the

Setting and achieving goals can really boost your self-esteem.

Ensure that your goals are achievable and that you are not setting yourself up for a failure in order feed your lack of self-esteem.

steps on the way to get there and celebrate the small victories as it's unlikely to happen overnight. It can also be helpful to write down the successes you have already experienced. Sometimes when you're going through a difficult period and your goals seem out of reach it's important to know that you have achieved in the past. Success *is* a transferable skill

Try writing down your successes to remind yourself of them when you're going through a difficult period.

2. Dealing with your own inner critic. Most of us are completely unaware of how harshly we treat ourselves as we're so conditioned to our habitual thought patterns. Try and become aware of the 'running commentary' you play in your own head. Can you catch yourself berating yourself? Would you speak to a friend, colleague or loved one in that way? Try to consciously replace a negative focus with the positives in a situation. This doesn't mean ignoring problems, it means dealing with them head on while simultaneously praising yourself and others for what is working. If you find it hard to 'catch' your inner thoughts, try and find some time to write down, unedited, how you are feeling. If you do it regularly, without censoring yourself, you may pick up on negative themes

Many of us are far harsher on ourselves than we would be with other people.

Would you speak to a friend, colleague or loved one in that way? How would you react if someone else spoke to you in that manner?

If you find it difficult to 'catch' your critical inner monologue, try and find some time to write down, unedited, how you are feeling.

3. Learning to relax. We live in such a 'doing' culture it can be hard to find ways to switch off. If we don't schedule in regular relaxation activities, we can go too far when we finally let go (such as binge drinking or comfort eating). What makes you feel happy? A trip to the cinema? A good book? A drink with a friend? Regardless of how senior you are in your organisation, you need to make room for leisure in your life. We are human beings as well as human doings

   Relaxation and switching off from the stresses and worries of life can help self-esteem.

   Think about what makes you happy and what would relax you, then make the time to do these things.

4. Looking after yourself. This means staying healthy, eating good quality food and taking some form of exercise. Eat better and move more. We all know these principles but it can be very easy to find excuses to ignore them

   Try to look after yourself through healthy eating and exercise.

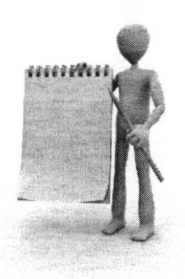

Exercises

A very quick and effective way to see if messages from your childhood are affecting your self-esteem is to write the following headings in your notebook and jot down the answers:

- Things my mother used to say to me about life/myself

- Things my father used to say to me about life/myself

- Things other authority figures used to say (such as teachers, clergymen, other influential adults)

Do you recognise any of your current thinking in your responses? Is that the way you would think if you had a choice?

Gratitude list. It can be easy to focus on what we don't have in our professional and personal life to the detriment of what we do. Write down in your notebook 20 things you are grateful for in your life. Repeat this exercise regularly – doing this makes us happier, more relaxed and, ironically, more open to getting what may currently be out of our reach.

Affirmations. Choose a situation you would like to be in or a quality you would like to possess. Then write down or say your statement as if it is already true, e.g. "I am a caring and compassionate leader", "I inspire respect and motivation in my team" or "I am a worthwhile person". It can feel silly at first, but try and push past your internal resistance and continue. A lot of our current, unconscious affirmations are formed from years of negative self-talk. Once you are aware of the ways you talk down to yourself, try and reformulate the phrases in the positive and keep repeating them. Choose something that feels relevant and repeat until it feels true. The brain can take a while to get used to the new 'reality', but this is a really effective exercise if you stick with it.

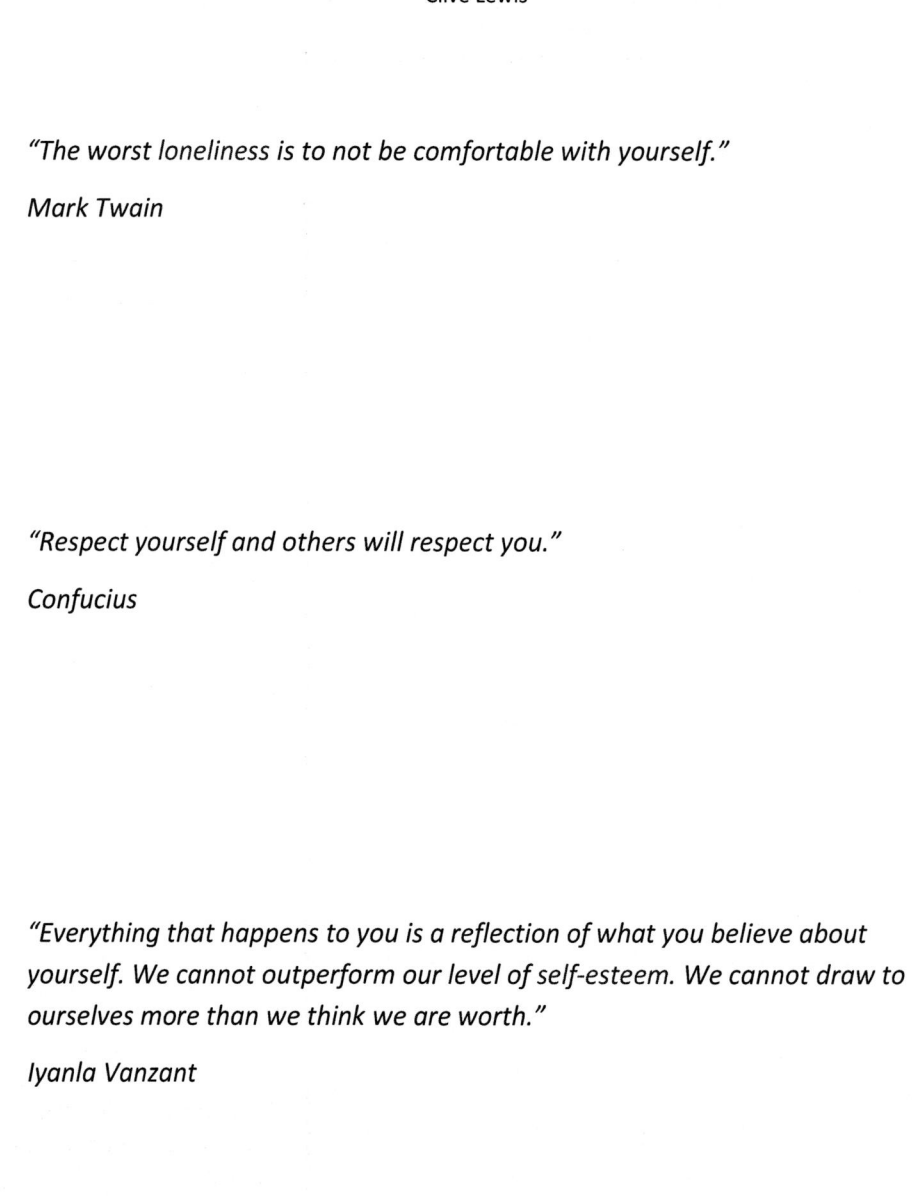

"The worst loneliness is to not be comfortable with yourself."

Mark Twain

"Respect yourself and others will respect you."

Confucius

"Everything that happens to you is a reflection of what you believe about yourself. We cannot outperform our level of self-esteem. We cannot draw to ourselves more than we think we are worth."

Iyanla Vanzant

Chapter Nine: Actions speak loudest

A lot of words have been spoken and a lot of trees felled to create the reports and recommendations following the numerous inquiries into the UK healthcare sector. You may have given a talk to your organisation or team about the need to improve compassion and care within the culture. But, in order to avoid the accusation of lip service, your words need to be translated into meaningful action.

Reports, recommendations and enquiries are all well and good, but these need to be followed by definitive, meaningful action.

We all know how it feels to be on the receiving end of empty promises or great plans that somehow never see the light of day. We can feel let down, mistrustful, and unwilling to put our faith in that person again, however inspiring or exciting their next project appears. To avoid falling into that trap, keep the following principles in mind.

Empty promises or encouraging plans that never see the light of day can dent our faith in future projects or individuals.

Go the extra mile

It always feels good when you know that someone has gone out of their way to help you out. You feel valued, appreciated, and your faith in humanity is upheld. It also feels good to be that person and extend yourself in service of another human being. It's a virtuous circle.

When you know that someone has gone out of their way to help you it helps restore your faith in humanity, as well as giving you a positive view of that person.

We do, however, live in the real world where we need to carry out our jobs efficiently and effectively, and there simply aren't enough hours in the day to do this with *every* patient or team member, *every* time. But calling to make sure someone has got home safely, staying for a chat with a patient who doesn't have any visitors, spending a bit more time with a patient's family to explain the implications of treatment and how it may affect them as well as the individual – all these things are noticed and appreciated.

Huge gestures aren't always possible or indeed the best use of one's time, but think back to the Richard Branson letter – even if you haven't time to put pen to paper, a quick phone call to make sure a patient got back safely can make a huge difference.

These days, time is one of the scarcest resources in healthcare (particularly in the NHS), and therefore the most valuable. Making it possible for your team to spend more time with their patients and their families could be the single most effective thing you can do in helping to bring about a more compassionate culture within your organisation.

Time is a valuable commodity, so making it possible for your team to spend as much of it with patients and families illustrates where your priorities lie, both to patients and your team.

Information, information, information

One of the most frustrating aspects about being a patient in a hospital or other healthcare setting is the enforced passivity and powerlessness. Other people are making decisions about your treatment, and you can feel reduced to a number on a set of notes, or an

As a patient, a lack of information is one of the most frustrating things.

appointment time, which is a very dehumanising experience.

One way you can help patients is to give them as much information about their condition or situation as possible, along with a plan of treatment, if appropriate. In Chapter Seven we looked at how 'information overload' makes your team and organisation less effective. This however, is different. Providing patients with information about their condition, about possible outcomes, treatment options, etc. actively demonstrates care. People want to be empowered to make decisions about their health, and giving them plenty of information acknowledges that.

Make sure your team is as clued-up as they can be about treatment and conditions so they can, in turn, pass on this knowledge to patients. Have plenty of printed material available as people may be too overwhelmed to take in all the information offered at a consultation or on the ward, and will want to digest it at home with more space and time.

Say sorry

Some people are fearful of apologising because they think it will make them look bad, or weak. But we are all imperfect, and there is no shame in revealing this to

One way you can help is to ensure that your team provides as much information to patients as is appropriate in a timely manner.

People want to be empowered to make decisions about their health, and giving them plenty of information acknowledges that.

Make sure your team is as clued-up as they can be about treatment and conditions so they can, in turn, pass on this knowledge to patients.

Some people see apologising as a show of weakness, but if anything it is the opposite – a show of security in who we are.

others if we feel secure enough in our own skin. Even the little things count. If a patient has been kept waiting, the very first thing they will want to hear is, "I'm sorry". If you arrive late or have to cancel a one to one meeting with a staff member, apologise. If you have made a mistake in a report for your chief executive, acknowledge it. There will be plenty of opportunities for explaining the whys and wherefores after, but admitting when you've slipped up can help build bridges and, ironically, improve team morale. If you find yourself having to apologise a lot, you will have to look into the reasons you're making so many mistakes/inconveniencing the other person, but the effort should be put into remedying this, not reducing the number of times you say sorry.

A patient who has been put out in some way wants to hear you start with "I'm sorry", regardless of the scale of the problem.

If you find yourself having to apologise numerous times then there could be something procedurally wrong in your department that warrants investigation.

Of course, in cases of medical negligence, there may be legal issues that prevent an individual or organisation taking ownership of the blame, but in general, if a mistake has been made, own up.

Express your gratitude

This may sound obvious, but how often do you really appreciate someone's effort or attitude? People like to be thanked and to know that they have made a difference. If you're not in the habit of actively appreciating your team, go out of your way to notice

People like to be thanked and to know that they have made a difference, but it can sometimes become too easy to stop thanking people.

something they have done, or a quality that they have, and make it sincere. It may seem a little forced at first if you're not used to it, but identifying positive actions and showing your gratitude will encourage more of the same.

It may seem unusual but try and thank (or encourage your frontline staff to thank) the patients too. We're used to the healthcare practitioner being thanked for their efforts, but a "thank you for waiting", "thank you for understanding" or "thank you for changing your appointment at such short notice" also goes a long way.

Encourage the use of expressing gratitude in your team, and even to patients.

Actively prioritise

When our time and attention are in great demand, we need to focus on what is *really* important. One of the most effective actions we can take that shows we're putting our money where our mouth is, is to identify our top priorities and either delegate or disregard everything else. Ask yourself, "if care and compassion were the principles guiding my work today, what would I do first, and what would seem less important?" This principle should work for people at all levels of seniority within an organisation. If it doesn't matter, don't do it. Encourage your staff to do the same - if they're not

Identify your top priorities and either delegate or disregard everything else.

Allow yourself to be guided by the twin lights of 'care' and 'compassion' in prioritisation.

sure, they can always check with you. But keep revising your list.

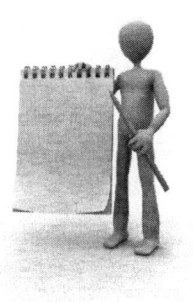

Exercises

Where can you translate words into action? Complete the following sentences in your notebook:

- "If our organisation really cared about its staff and patients, it would..."
- "If I really cared about my team, I would..."
- "If my team really cared about their patients, they would..."

Then do it!

"I have always thought the actions of men the best interpreters of their thoughts."

John Locke

"Well done is better than well said."

Benjamin Franklin

"Action is the antidote to despair."

Joan Baez

Chapter Ten: Patients as customers

For some people, the concept of customer service in a healthcare setting can seem inappropriate, as if the patient-clinician relationship can be reduced to a simple "transaction". Consider the idea in more depth, and you will discover that a commitment to improving patient experience and attention to detail makes a huge difference to patients and employees alike.

The concept of 'customer service' in a healthcare setting can sometimes be seen as inappropriate, but when considered in more depth the notion is a very pertinent one.

It is not overly radical to suggest that a patient's stay in your premises, however short or long, should be as comfortable and stress-free as possible. Unfortunately, at least in the NHS, the reality falls far short of that ideal. A 2009 survey of 337 NHS Chief Executives and Chairs found that 100% felt that the NHS wasn't customer-focused, and 65% of those believed a "significant change" was required[16]. This concern was echoed by the general public, 93% of whom felt that the NHS needed to pay more attention to customer service. Areas for improvement included:

A patient's stay in your premises should be as comfortable and stress-free as possible.

A 2009 survey revealed that an overwhelming number of executives felt that NHS customer service was far below expectations.

- Friendlier staff
- Easier appointment booking systems
- Clearer information about treatment
- Better bedside manner

Only 7% of the general public disagreed with this finding.

Attending a healthcare setting, particularly for a surgical procedure or in an acute care situation, can be traumatic for the patient and their family. Imagine if you could enhance their experience by making improvements in all of the above areas?

Great customer service is also becoming more of a priority on a national scale. Reports in May 2013 showed A&E attendances were up 50% on the previous decade. The resources of the NHS are already squeezed and there is much that is out of the individual Trust's (or senior manager's) control. So it makes sense to make changes where you can, invest in customer care that goes beyond glossy posters or slogans on leaflets, and make a genuine difference to everyone who uses or provides your services.

Where do you stand on customer service?

Do you have a customer service charter? If you do, can you honestly say, hand on heart, that you live it to the letter? Below is an example from The Royal Marsden, giving top line standards for which all staff are accountable, every day[17].

Throughout all contact with customers, staff should aim to meet their needs through professional, courteous and efficient service. Staff will:

Attending a healthcare setting can be traumatic for the patient and their family. You can help make a difference in all areas of this experience.

NHS resources are already squeezed and there is much that is out of control of the individual Trust's (or senior manager's) control.

Investing in proper customer care can make a genuine difference to everyone who uses or provides your services.

Few of us can honestly say that we fully live up to a customer service charter, should one be in place.

- Treat all customers with respect and courtesy
- Listen to what customers have to say
- Personalise services to the needs and circumstances of each service user where practical
- Always do what they say they are going to do, or update the appropriate people promptly if things change, offering an explanation for the change
- Respond to enquiries promptly and efficiently
- Consult customers about their service needs

These standards are applicable to telephone etiquette, website availability, face to face meetings, cover for colleagues, training, consultation and feedback, and monitoring of customer service levels.

Such standards are applicable to all situations, from telephone conversations to training sessions.

The areas on which you need to focus your customer service attention will vary, but the following should be covered as a minimum:

A friendly demeanour
A warm smile towards patients is one of the most basic tenets of customer service, and yet a staggering number of people overlook it. In a healthcare setting, where emotions run high and patients and their families may be anxious about treatment, a reassuring

Maintaining a warm, pleasant attitude is not always easy in stressful situations, but you should try to remember the reassuring power of a simple smile at all times.

smile goes a long way. This principle should apply to all staff, regardless of seniority. Managers can set a good example by being friendly and approachable with their teams as well as visitors to the organisation.

Managers can set a good example by treating teams and visitors with this attitude.

Speedy communication

Whether contact is by phone, email or via social media, you should try to set minimum waiting times for your responses. In the private sector, many companies have a "five second maximum" response to answering telephones, and a 24-hour limit for emails. One of the major complaints of people calling hospitals or other healthcare providers is phones ringing endlessly, or being put through to department after department. If you know you will be out of the office, give people the opportunity to leave you a voicemail message, but make sure you return the call as promptly as possible.

Try to set minimum waiting times for communication in all mediums.

We all know what it's like to be placed eternally on hold or batted from one department to another, so try and avoid this in your department.

There are often staffing issues within the NHS (which have an impact on response times) but you need to be able to meet the commitments you make. If you regularly have to set your voicemail because no one in the department is available, how can you address this? Is it as simple as staggering break and lunchtimes, or do you need to look at deploying more staff at peak times? Details like this may seem relatively minor in the grand scheme of things, but are actually incredibly important

Consider the issue from all points of view, from small scale to large scale.

to patients who may not be able to keep calling back at your convenience.

Computer says "no"

Unwieldy, bureaucratic organisations are frustrating for those who work in them as well as for their customers. One way to humanise your processes is to give frontline employees the freedom to exercise their judgment in customer service situations. When people are constrained by their role and treated like robots with little autonomy, they are more likely to act in a similar way towards the customer.

Giving employees autonomy is a good way to improve interaction between staff and patients.

Receptionists should have the freedom to make decisions about queues. Nurses need to be able to give the parent of a sick child a sandwich if they have no change for the vending machine. Staff should not face reprisals if they are responding to a customer service need in a helpful and proportionate way. They are also likely to perform well and act in a caring manner when they feel trusted to use their discretion. Even in an organisation as "standardised" as the NHS, employees need to feel they can help the person in front of them, rather than constantly having to refer back to a supervisor. As David Freemantle says, in his book *Incredible Customer Service*[18], "the people who know

Bureaucracy should not prevent staff acting in ways that suppress their natural desire to help those who need it most.

the customers best should have as much responsibility as possible for pleasing them".

Customer service within your team

When you prioritise excellent customer service in your organisation, everyone becomes a customer. This means treating your staff with the same courtesy you would extend to a patient or family member. Make sure their surroundings are as comfortable as those for "outsiders" - i.e. clean toilets, well-equipped staffrooms and quick responses to internal enquiries.

Training

In order to get your team onside, you need someone to show them how to apply principles of great customer service to their daily work in a way that is relevant and motivating. All too often, managers bring in expensive consultants who have little appreciation of the participants' actual jobs, teaching all sorts of theoretical ideas that would work brilliantly in a different organisation but which are wholly impractical in, say, a care home or GP surgery.

The NHS Next Stage Review[19] states: "the skills for listening, understanding and responding to the needs of individual patients and supporting them to manage their health in a manner that is respectful of diversity

"The people who know the customers best should have as much responsibility as possible for pleasing them."

Treat your staff with the same courtesy you would extend to a patient or family member.

Allow everyone to become a customer, staff included.

Customer service consultants can perform a service, but their theories are often ill suited to, say, a small GP surgery.

and difference must, wherever possible, be incorporated into education and training programmes."

To ensure your training programme is more than hot air and actually makes your team want to go out and apply these principles, ask for recommendations and see which trainers have been successfully used by other Trusts or healthcare organisations.

Feedback

How do you feel about customer feedback? Is it something you fear or welcome? A commitment to good customer service means addressing every bit of feedback you receive, by the person to whom it is addressed, in a timely fashion. If the chief executive receives a letter of complaint, he or she should answer it personally, likewise the director of nursing or individual healthcare professional. If there are too many complaints for the CEO to handle, it is this issue that needs to be tackled, rather than quibbling about who answers the post. People want to know that their voices have been genuinely heard, and no standardised, generic response will do that.

Canvas your team for trainer recommendations – this will help ensure that your training programme gets your team involved.

A commitment to good customer service means facing the bad feedback as well as enjoying the good.

Letters addressed to individuals within an organisation should be answered by that person and not palmed off to a customer service team.

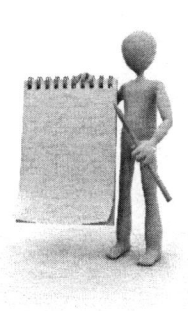

Exercises

Do you have a Customer Service or Customer Care Charter? If not, have a look at those created by similar organisations and create one that is meaningful, realistic and inspirational.

If you do have one (or once you have established one), review each section and score yourself out of ten for where you think you are now.

Identify your top three worst performing areas and address these first. What changes can you make (or persuade others to make)? Is it a case of ensuring vending machines are stocked and the magazines available at reception are regularly renewed, or do you need to look at more complex issues such as staffing?

Involve your team along the way. Everyone needs to be on board when it comes to creating excellent customer service. You need to sell the benefits to the employees before they will be felt by patients. Write down in your notebook, "Ten reasons why improving customer service will make XXX a better place to visit and to work" and brainstorm some ideas. The more everyone understands the benefits, as well as the strategic importance, of delivering excellent service, the more likely they are to provide it, day after day.

"If you work just for the money, you'll never make it, but if you love what you're doing and always put the customer first, success will be yours."

Ray Kroc, Founder of McDonald's

"We see our customers as invited guests to a party and we are the hosts. It's our job every day to make every important aspect of the customer experience a little bit better."

Jeff Bezos, CEO, Amazon.com

"Our mission statement about treating people with respect and dignity is not just words but a creed we live by every day. You can't expect your employees to exceed the expectations of your customers if you don't exceed the employees' expectations of management."

Howard Schultz, CEO, Starbucks

Chapter Eleven: Culture shift

What is organisational culture?

Ask the average worker about their company's culture, and they'll probably describe it in terms of the CEO's or founder's style, e.g. "it's fun and relaxed and very family-friendly", or "it's pretty serious and full-on but people are rewarded for their hard work and loyalty". Managers tend to hire people who are like themselves (not the best managers, I hasten to add), which perpetuates the cultural style. So entrenched is the average organisation's culture that it can take a dramatic event, such as a significant loss of sales or a scandal (such as the NHS care home inquiries in 2012/13), to prompt change.

Managers tend to hire people who are like themselves, which perpetuates the cultural style.

It can take a dramatic event to change some organisations' cultures.

Cultural issues within the healthcare sector

Although more common in the NHS than private healthcare organisations, some of the themes I regularly encounter include:

- An inflexible, hierarchical employment structure
- A bureaucratic ethos

- Poor communication between managers and frontline staff, leading to a "them and us" attitude

- Stressed and overworked employees

- Entrenched attitudes about "how things are done"

Of course, I am deliberately focusing on the negative areas, as the focus of this chapter is "change". Please bear in mind if you recognise your workplace in the above description that a) you are not alone and b) there is something you can do about it!

How would you define your working culture?

The best way to get a handle on your particular organisation's culture is to spend a day looking at it as if you were an outsider. Take notes on everything – how it looks physically (outside and internal decor, noticeboards, posters, etc), how people interact with each other, the type of conversation you might overhear, etc. How do people talk to each other? What are people saying (or indeed not saying)? For example, you might claim to place the patient at the heart of your activities, but if you don't engage in or overhear a single

Look at your organisation as if you were an outsider.

How does it look, how do people interact, what types of conversations do you overhear?

If you don't engage your organisation from a patient's point of view, you can't hope to change it for their benefit.

conversation about the patient experience in a day's work, this is very telling.

In your next few team meetings, ask some informal questions about it. By asking "how would you describe this place to a friend in three words?", you'll get a pretty accurate picture of the culture. Another quick fire way of determining your culture is to identify the person you think of as a "typical" employee. What are these typical qualities or traits?

Ask your team the same questions and see how their opinions match with yours.

Where do you want to go?

Culture, according to a dictionary definition, is all about "customs, ideas and values". This can seem a bit vague and wishy washy until you really pin it down. How would you *like* your friend to describe your place of work? In order to move in the right direction, you need to be clear about where you want to go. Painting a picture of your ideal work culture should feel exciting and inspiring. Is this picture at odds with your current reality? In what ways? Choose a couple of themes that stand out and use these as your starting point.

You need to have an image of how you would like others to see your organisation, from which you can start to paint a picture of the culture.

Stand your ideal culture up against the existing culture and choose the most glaring mismatches to start from.

Author of *The Wall Street Guide to Management*[20], Alan Murray, offers his top tips for kickstarting culture change:

- Start the change process with people who have disproportionate influence in the organisation

- Look for ways to get people to experience the harsh realities that make change necessary

How could you implement these two points into your own culture change exercise? Firstly, identify those who have "disproportionate influence". This usually includes the CEO and senior management team, but may also include others whose opinions hold a lot of credibility among the workforce, such as a union representative. If the organisation is large enough, you will also have an internal communications team to support you and provide creative input. Don't worry about getting everyone onside at once, but start at the top and slowly work your way down. You might discover that the chief executive is so inspired by your changes that you have no further work to do to convince the other "influencers"!

Identify those in your department or organisation who have "disproportionate influence" (a CEO or senior management team for example) and sound them out about your ideas for change.

Alan Murray's second suggestion about getting people to "experience the harsh realities that make change necessary" is crucial to make sure your campaign has longevity and that senior staff *really* understand why change is necessary. How can those at the top know how it really feels to be a harassed staff nurse pulled in too many directions at once? Or what the receptionist has to put up with from disgruntled patients who have been waiting over an hour for their appointment? By doing it themselves. Encouraging management to spend real, quality time (at least a day, regularly) on the "shop floor" is a vital intelligence gathering exercise for them (as well as good internal PR for the organisation). It will also make your job a lot easier to persuade them of the need for a culture change.

Encouraging management to spend real, quality time (at least a day, regularly) on the "shop floor" is a vital intelligence gathering exercise for them (as well as good internal PR for the organisation).

Murray also makes the following suggestions:

- Establish mixed taskforce teams. When working on team projects, the principle of "like attracts like" may predominate. Try to proactively mix people up, ensuring a good mix of age, gender and experience

- Change the physical environment. Get rid of "exclusive" office suites and place people in closer physical proximity to each other, regardless of their position in the hierarchy

- Foster flexibility where possible. Employees like to feel valued and trusted. They also like to have a sense of control over their working lives, so offer them as many opportunities as possible to do this. Can you offer some flexible hours, or home working? Obviously, this is not possible within some shift patterns (at hospitals, for example), but within every role there should be some room for manoeuvre

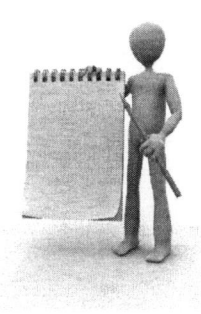

Exercises

After spending a day "observing", write down in a paragraph or less how you would define your organisation's culture.

Now write down how you would ideally like it to be. What are the main areas of difference?

Who are the people with the largest influence within your organisation? Who would you feel most comfortable sharing your vision with?

Does your organisation already have staff on the "shop floor"? If not, it is a really important exercise for senior managers to undertake. What do you need to do to start the ball rolling? Who do you need to talk to? What do you need to say to them to convince them?

Examine the areas for "quick wins". What is within your power to change? Where can the physical environment be more comfortable and relaxed for employees and patients? How can you give others a greater sense of control over their lives while they're in the building? Smaller scale changes can often be the catalyst for something bigger, so don't overlook the details.

"Change is hard because people overestimate the value of what they have – and underestimate the value of what they may gain by giving that up."

James Belasco and Ralph Stayer

"There is nothing more difficult to take in hand, more perilous to conduct, or more uncertain in its success, than to take the lead in the introduction of a new order of things."

Machiavelli

"People don't resist change. They resist being changed!"

Peter Senge

Clive Lewis

Chapter Twelve: A note on saying sorry

"Being involved in an adverse medical event can be a devastating experience for care providers."[21]

Some of you reading that statement may well be able to relate, and whilst errors in surgical procedure are often cited when discussing negligence in the medical field, there are situations when all of us must apologise for errors made in our professional lives. Patient care, at all levels, can be a complicated journey with numerous difficult decisions to make, ranging from which medication to administer to what kind of care is most suitable for the patient. Hopefully you and your team will get all the calls right, but the law of averages says that on some occasions you won't. When things do go wrong it is important to know how to go about dealing with the situation in the right way.

When things go wrong, it is important to apologise honestly, quickly and without reservation. Apologising allows both sides to begin to draw a line under an episode that will, in all likelihood, have been very distressing for all concerned and may have been progressing or escalating for a while. It will allow you to continue with your career and learn from your mistakes rather than constantly justifying your case, possibly to

There are situations when all of us must apologise for errors made in our professional lives.

Healthcare can be a delicate, complicated industry and mistakes will naturally happen.

When things do go wrong it is important to know how to go about dealing with the situation in the right way.

Apologising allows both sides to begin to draw a line under a potentially distressing episode for the patient and their loved ones.

the courts as well as to yourself and associates and employers. If you were genuinely at fault, it is important to admit this as soon as possible and to try to move on.

The power and importance of apology is something that is often overlooked by those who have made an honest mistake. In Michigan, the hospitals in the University health system have seen annual legal fees drop from $3m to $1m following the adoption of a policy to openly admit and apologise for surgical mistakes, while notices of intent to sue have more than halved[22]. We have all been in situations where mistakes have been made to our detriment, and it is no overstatement to say that even large-scale errors can be greatly smoothed over with a genuine, heartfelt and speedy apology. Quite simply, we want to know that the person or company that made the error cares about what happened to us, even if the damage is irreparable.

Apologising is more complicated than you might think, especially for those who find it difficult to admit guilt. The following steps outline what apologies should contain and how to go about conducting these specific kinds of difficult conversations.

Providing it comes from the heart, a simple "I'm sorry" has immense power, but it is something that a surprising amount of people overlook, perhaps feeling that it is

If you were genuinely at fault, it is important to admit this as soon as possible, learn from the mistakes made, and to try and move on.

The power of apology is something that is often overlooked by those who have made an honest mistake.

We have all been in situations where mistakes have been made to our detriment, and even large-scale errors can be greatly smoothed over with a genuine, heartfelt and speedy apology.

Apologising is more complicated than you might think, especially for those not naturally disposed to taking blame.

inadequate in certain circumstances. This short phrase, however, is so effective because it provides no excuses or caveats, it doesn't deflect blame and it gets right to the point. It may sound simplistic, but this is the first thing you should say when apologising to someone, and you should say it concisely and with the appropriate corresponding body language (constant eye contact and a subdued posture, for example). It should be kept short and meaningful before moving onto the next stage. For those who feel that 'sorry' may not be enough, phrases such as 'you have my unreserved apology' could also be considered.

The next stage, that of accepting responsibility, is, as many doctors will know, a very tricky area to navigate. Patients will want to hear that you accept responsibility for whatever mistakes were made, but it is inadvisable to admit directly to patients which individuals were responsible for which areas of failure. Instead, it is better for a healthcare professional to use phrases along the lines of "I am very sorry for the decisions that were taken". As you can see, this admits culpability but doesn't negatively affect your legal standing. The patient may want more than this, but try and avoid admitting personal guilt to any one decision or area, or mentioning names of others and their part in events.

Ensure that you start with an 'I'm sorry'. This short phrase is so effective because it provides no excuses or caveats, it doesn't deflect blame and it gets right to the point.

Say it concisely with the corresponding apologetic body language.

For those who feel that 'sorry' may not be enough, phrases such as 'you have my unreserved apology' could also be considered.

Accepting responsibility is a tricky area to navigate for healthcare professionals.

It is inadvisable to admit directly to patients which individuals were responsible for which areas of failing.

Admitting culpability makes us doubt our self-worth, and no one likes to be considered a failure, but this step is very important.

The next stage of your apology depends on the circumstances. Each individual case is different, and you should take cues from the patient or their representative, but further explanation of the mistake will often be required. This is usually nothing to do with the patient or their representative wanting to 'punish' you, it is simply human nature to want an explanation when something has gone wrong – we want to know why certain things were said or done, who made those decisions and why. Don't go into details if they don't ask, but be prepared to honestly explain your actions if required, again adding that you are very sorry for the wrong decisions taken.

The next stage centres on your desire to make amends. This will depend largely on the current situation – if a patient has passed away then there is very little you will be able to do, but hopefully there will still be time in which to act. The key here is to ask what you can do to help, not tell the patient/representatives what you intend to do for them; the former indicates that you are willing to listen to what they think is suitable recompense, whilst the latter suggests you have already equated their grief and anguish to a task you can perform. An act of contrition can also help provide a sense of closure for the patient/their loved ones. A trap

The following step depends on the demands of the patient, but often an explanation will be required.

Again, as far as possible do not deflect blame. Don't go into details unless requested by the patient – keep it honest, heartfelt and concise.

Following this should be an offer to make amends.

In some cases where the patient has passed away there may not be much you can do except learn a lesson for next time.

Ensure that you ask the patient's representatives what they would like you to do for them, rather than telling them what you will offer to do.

to avoid here, however, is to overpromise in order to placate them. You need to be honest and state what you can and can't deliver, and hopefully a reasonable compromise can be sought.

Be honest with your capabilities – don't promise what you can't deliver purely to placate the other party.

Just like all difficult conversations, apologies themselves do not always go to plan. You may be faced with a range of emotions, demands and even threats, and sometimes all you have to offer is a wall of apologies. It can feel a little defeating at times to say the least, but never underestimate the power of a genuine apology – if conducted in the right way it can not only have the short-term benefit of calming agitated individuals but it has also been shown to reduce the likelihood of further action by patients or their representatives. It may even help you to sleep better at night.

You may be faced with a range of emotions, demands and even threats, and sometimes all you have to offer is a wall of apologies.

It can feel a little defeating at times to say the least, but never underestimate the power of a genuine apology when the dust has settled.

It is also important to ensure that a mistake is not just addressed, but, more importantly, that it is learnt from. There are various ways of doing this, but one increasingly popular method is via an 'After Action Report', or AAR. The website Knowledge Sharing Toolkit defines an AAR as "a simple process used by a team to capture the lessons learned from past successes and failures, with the goal of improving future performance." It encourages participants to discuss honestly and openly

A mistake should not just be addressed, but also learnt from.

Consider using an After Action Report (AAR) to analyse performance and highlight areas for improvement.

how an event or process went/is progressing and outlines potential areas of improvement.

An AAR doesn't just help to analyse and correct a mistake that has been made; it can also be used to evaluate any event or system/process in order to improve performance, whether successful or otherwise. I have provided a link[23] in the references section of this book to an online AAR toolkit, but a quick internet search will allow you to find other resources on AARs, including other methods of conducting them that may be more suitable to your particular organisation, department or team.

An AAR can be used to evaluate any event or system/process in order to improve performance, whether successful or otherwise.

Chapter Thirteen: Keep at it!

If the road to Hell is paved with good intentions, how do you maintain your enthusiasm and motivation for bringing about change? The fact that you have picked up this book in the first place and read this far demonstrates that you are genuinely committed to improving compassion, care and respect within your organisation. But how can you sustain that engagement in the face of time pressures, institutional challenges and the daily grind, not to mention resistance you may meet from within your team, or from your own managers?

The fact you have got this far shows that you at least have the motivation to attempt change, but keeping it going is another challenge.

Chart your progress

It's time to revisit the goals you wrote down in your notebook at the end of Chapter One. How are they going? What about the habits you decided to adopt after reading Chapter Three? You don't need to have completed every single task to acknowledge how far you've come – just chipping away on a regular basis can be a huge achievement. How you choose to celebrate or reward yourself for these achievements is up to you, but don't let success pass unnoticed. Attaining your goals can be a heady feeling, and you may be tempted to rush straight into making new ones. Of course it's

How are you doing in working towards your goals of Chapter One?

What about the habits from Chapter Three?

Attaining goals, no matter how small, can lead to further success, so enjoy them and move on!

important to maintain momentum, but make sure you give yourself a metaphorical pat on the back for the work you've put in so far.

Stay accountable

Whether or not you adopted a formal mentoring system as discussed in Chapter Four, it can be helpful to share your achievements with another person to keep you on course. You might have chosen to be discreet about your work until now, but if you have something concrete to show for your time and efforts, why not involve a co-worker or a manager? They may have noticed the change in atmosphere or improvement in patient feedback without being aware of the source.

Having the involvement of another colleague or more senior manager offers the added benefit of potentially doubling your resources and reach – you may well be able to achieve more things in the future with colleagues who are on side. Why not suggest to your manager that you give him or her an update on your progress at your regular one to ones? Their enthusiasm for your vision may take it to places you never imagined at the start of your journey.

Sharing your achievements can also boost your morale and give you encouragement to move onto further success.

Colleagues may have noticed a change in you and may want to know how you did it!

The involvement of others within your team/wider organisation has the benefit of doubling your resources and reach.

You will be able to judge the environment and people involved with regard to spreading the word.

Become part of the bigger picture

Making tangible progress can give you confidence to reach out to like minded individuals. What are people in other Trusts or organisations doing to embed care and compassion within their culture? How can your work become part of something regional or even nationwide? Whether you make contact while networking at an industry event or get in touch with someone who has published their work online, don't hide your light under the proverbial bushel. Your ideas could be just what someone else is looking for, and vice versa. Offer to give a talk to your team – maybe one day you might be addressing a whole conference about your work. Sometimes it takes an impassioned speech to jolt us out of our routine activities and thoughts. Step up and be that person.

What are people in other trusts or organisations doing to embed care and compassion within their culture?

How can your work become part of something regional or even nationwide?

Don't hide your success away – your ideas could be just what someone else is looking for.

Keep your vision in mind

What was that single event or idea you had that made you pick up this book? Was it an absence of something, a feeling, or maybe a conversation? Was it positive or negative? Has it changed since you started out? You might want to choose an object to symbolise your vision (no one needs to know what it represents other than you) and keep it on your desk or at home. When you appreciate that each step you take will bring you closer

Keep in mind the factors that motivated you to pick up this book in the first place.

You may wish to have them easily accessible in case your motivation dips.

to achieving your vision, it will be easier to maintain enthusiasm and drive.

Keeping a visual reminder somewhere is also great for getting your subconscious to work on your plan while you're busy with other things. It could be a note from a patient who was appreciative of your team having gone the extra mile or, conversely, a copy of a government inquiry into poor care. Some people are more motivated by avoiding the repetition of something bad than actively moving towards a positive image. Experiment until you find something that, when you look at it, makes you itch to spring into action.

You may find that some form of a visual reminder helps – perhaps a letter from a patient, or a note about the success of yourself or your team.

See one, do one, teach one

Often the best way of integrating something into our experience is to explain it to someone else. As the saying goes, "we teach what we most need to learn". Why not assimilate some of your learnings into your team's workplan? Choose the exercises that have resonated most with you from this book and share them with your team. The degree to which you formalise this is entirely up to you, but sharing some of your favourite techniques will cement them in your mind and inspire others. You may wish to lend them a copy of this book

Why not try to assimilate some elements of this book into your team's workplan, for example exercises you found most successful. It can't hurt, and you may find that one success leads to more.

and ask them for their own ideas about practical ways to show compassion and respect within the workplace.

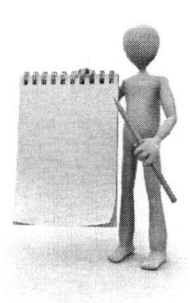

Exercises

Think about how you want to review your progress so far. Would a full 'report' on your actions be inspiring and motivating? Or would you prefer a bullet point 'highs and lows' approach? Either way, be sure to include the good, the bad and the ugly. Look at what worked, and what wasn't so effective. Why was one thing so successful and how could you build on it? What would you change about what wasn't so successful? Be honest with yourself so you can focus your time and energies in the right direction.

Do something every day to further your progress. Of course there will be many demands on your time, but you don't have to spend hours a day on your project. Just writing down a thought on a post-it or having a conversation with a colleague will keep you moving forward. Acknowledge it all and appreciate yourself for your efforts.

Keep your notebook alive as a tool to help you achieve your goals. If you fill it up, buy another, but don't throw anything away. This is the evidence that you are doing what you can to improve the situation. It is your record of the difference you are making. Treasure it.

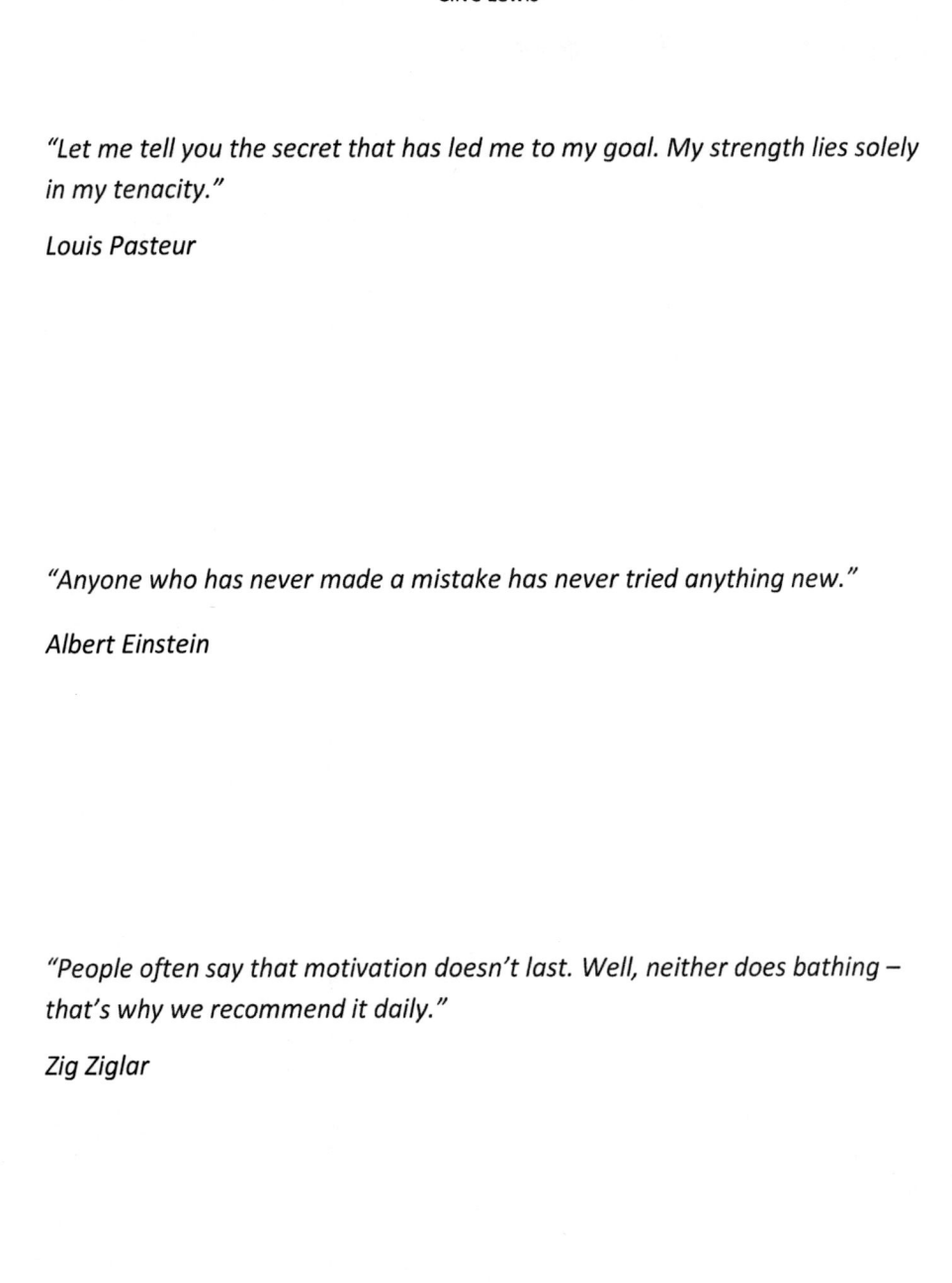

"Let me tell you the secret that has led me to my goal. My strength lies solely in my tenacity."

Louis Pasteur

"Anyone who has never made a mistake has never tried anything new."

Albert Einstein

"People often say that motivation doesn't last. Well, neither does bathing – that's why we recommend it daily."

Zig Ziglar

Conclusion

Congratulations for getting this far! I hope what you have read has been motivating and useful, and that you have already begun to implement some of the actions you identified in the last chapter.

Have you noticed any difference to your everyday work life as a result of completing the exercises? In particular, I hope you feel more passionate about your job, more aware of the difference you can make, and more connected to your team. As a result, you should feel more in control of your life, both in the workplace and in your personal interactions.

You may also discover that you are more effective and productive in your work. Too many people equate taking care of people as somehow 'time wasting' - and yet research points to compassionate leaders producing happier teams with reduced staff turnover, lower rates of sickness and less stress[24]. Managers who take the time to look after their staff and instil a compassionate culture within the workplace reap the dividends in business, as well as moral, terms. No one loses out.

The UK healthcare sector needs people like you, people who care enough to pick up a book like this and are prepared to make positive changes to improve their skills. If you found it helpful, please recommend it to your colleagues and friends. The more people who are committed to a caring, respectful and compassionate health service, the more we will all benefit by living healthier *and* happier lives.

Clive Lewis

About the author

Clive Lewis is a HR professional specialising in employee and industrial relations. He is a fellow of the Chartered Institute of Personnel and Development. His work has taken him across four continents. His handbook 'Difficult Conversations: 10 Steps to Becoming a Tackler not a Dodger' has been featured in The Sunday Times.

He serves as a non-executive director of an NHS Foundation Trust and virtual Board Member of NHS Employers. Much of his work is in the health sector.

He is heavily involved in charity work which provides mentoring, training and employability services for young males from poor socio-economic backgrounds. He was also the Chair of a Government appointed independent panel that produced the REACH report. The report identified a cost of underachievement to the UK economy of £24bn linked to this group.

Clive was awarded the OBE in 2011 and was commissioned as a Deputy Lieutenant in 2012.

Order form
Leadership with Compassion:
Applying Kindness, Dignity and Respect in Healthcare Management

Book Quantity	Price
1-14 copies	£9.99 each
15-29 copies	£7.99 each
30-99 copies	£5.99 each
100-999 copies	£5.75 each
1,000-4,999 copies	£5.50 each
5,000-9,999 copies	£5.25 each
10,000 or more copies	£5.00 each

Name: .... Job Title: ....

Organisation: ....

Address:...

Postcode: .... Tel No: ....

Email: ....

(Plus postage and packing – £3.00 per book)
☐ Cheque enclosed (Please make payable to Globis Ltd)
☐ Please invoice
☐ Please debit my credit card

Name on card: .... Card Number: ....

Start Date: .... Expiry Date: .... Security No: ....

Signed: ....

Post completed form to: Globis Ltd, Unit 1, Wheatstone Court, Quedgeley, Gloucester GL2 2AQ

Tel: 0330 100 0809
Email: info@globis.co.uk

References

1. The Sunday Times 100 Best Companies, 2013. *The Sunday Times*. [online] Available at: http://features.thesundaytimes.co.uk/public/best100companies/live/template [Accessed 10 June 2013].

2. *Tiny Habits*. [online] Available at: http://tinyhabits.com [Accessed 10 June 2013].

3. Covey, S. (1989). *The 7 Habits of Highly Effective People*. New York: Free Press.

4. *EMCC: Definitions for "Coaching" and "Mentoring"*. [online] Available at: http://www.emccouncil.org/webimages/CH/Aldo/Glossary_Coaching_Mentoring__EMCC_Switzerland_en_20.05.13.pdf [Accessed 24 September 2013].

5. *Institute of Healthcare Management*. [online] Available at: https://www.ihm.org.uk [Accessed 10 June 2013].

6. Harrold, F. (2006). *The Seven Rules of Success*. London: Hodder Paperbacks.

7. Bayley, H et al. (2004). *The Good Mentoring Toolkit for Healthcare*. Milton Keynes: Radcliffe Publishing Ltd.

8. Foster-Turner, J. (2005). *Coaching and Mentoring in Health and Social Care: The Essential Manual for Professionals and Organisations*. Milton Keynes: Radcliffe Publishing Ltd.

9. Ludwig, D.S., Kabat-Zinn, J. *Mindfulness in Medicine*. JAMA. 2008;300(11): 1350-1352.

10. Hutchinson, T.A., Dobkin, P.L. *Mindful Medical Practice: Just Another Fad?* Can Fam Physician. 2009 August; 55(8): 778–779.

11. Kabat-Zinn, J. (1994). *Wherever you go, there you are: Mindfulness meditation in everyday life*. New York: Hyperion Books.

12. West, M. (2012). Presentation entitled: *Workforce Resilience and Wellbeing for High Quality Care*.

13. Robertson Cooper i-resilience report. [online] Available at: http://www.robertsoncooper.com/iresilience/#.UkFmoGSbjNU [Accessed 24th September 2013].

14. *Be Mindful.* [online] Available at: http://bemindful.co.uk/ [Accessed 10 June 2013].

15. Coombes, F. (2012). *NLP Training In The NHS Workplace.* [online] Available at: http://www.positivehealth.com/article/nlp/nlp-training-in-the-nhs-workplace [Accessed 10 June 2013].

16. NHS (2009). *Customer Service in the NHS: Making Patient Care the Heart of Everything.* [online] Available at: http://www.you-unltd.co.uk/downloads/WhitePaper-CustomerServiceinNHSTrusts-Feb09.pdf [Accessed 10 June 2013].

17. The Royal Marsden (2010). *Customer Service Excellence – E-mail Response Audit.* [online] Available at: http://www.royalmarsden.nhs.uk/SiteCollectionDocuments/customer-service-excellence/customer-service-policy.pdf [Accessed 10 June 2013].

18. Freemantle, D. (1994). *Incredible Customer Service: The Final Test.* Maidenhead: McGraw-Hill Publishing Co.

19. Department of Health. (2008). *High Quality Care For All: NHS Next Stage Review Final Report (CM 7432).*

20. Murray, A. (2010). *The Wall Street Journal Essential Guide to Management: Lasting Lessons from the Best Leadership Minds of Our Time.* London: Harper Paperbacks.

21. MITSS. (2009). *MITSS for Clinicians.* [online] Available at: http://www.mitss.org/clinicians_home.html. [Accessed 10th June 2013].

22. Boothman, R.C., Blackwell, A.C., Campbell Jr, A.D., Commiskey, E and Anderson, S. *A Better Approach to Medical Malpractice Claims? The University of Michigan Experience.* JHLCL. 2009 January; 2(2): 125-159

23. *Knowledge Sharing Toolkit – After Action Report* [online] Available at: http://www.kstoolkit.org/After+Action+Review. [Accessed 24th September 2013].

24. Vianello, M., Galliani, E.M., and Haidt, J. *Elevation at work: The effects of leaders' moral excellence*. The Journal of Positive Psychology. 2010; 5(5): 390-411.

Leadership with Compassion: Applying Kindness, Dignity and Respect in Healthcare Management

Clive Lewis

Leadership with Compassion: Applying Kindness, Dignity and Respect in Healthcare Management

Clive Lewis